Efenians
The Book of Life

The Seven Noble Truths

JC PAULINO

EFENIANS

Efenians LLC

17350 State Highway 249 Ste 220

Houston, TX 77064

ISBN 978-1-7347841-0-7 (e-book)

ISBN 978-1-7347841-2-1 (paperback)

ISBN 978-1-7347841-1-4 (hardcopy)

Contact *www.efenians.com* with questions for the author or for discount information on bulk purchases.

With the utmost respect and admiration, I acknowledge the people who encouraged me to write this book and supported me throughout the whole process: my daughter Evelyn, my son Carlos, and my wife, Sofia. We gratefully acknowledge and express sincere appreciation to all those wonderful people who made this project possible.

To every child, born and unborn, who will inherit this planet and will make happiness their primary goal.

CONTENT

CONTENT

AUTHOR'S NOTE

Thank you for deciding to take this journey with me. You are about to go into a place where few people ever get to go and where fewer still will stay for long. I am referring to your internal place of peaceful and blissful tranquility, your quiet mind: the place where happiness resides, inside your evolved consciousness. We will explore a way of life, daily habits, and behaviors responsible for your holistic health and happiness. "Efenian's way"* is the name I have given this way of life. We will dive into why this is the only way to live if you want to experience the highest possible state of joy.

*Efe·nian: *noun:* Efenian; *plural noun* Efenians 1. One who is best version of you. 2. One committed to total mental and physical fitness.2. Inhabitants of Planet Fitness. 3. One who follows the Efenian's principles, of Efenian nature. 4. An optimally, holistically fit and happy individual. 5. A physically and mentally fit individual with a least a 90 **FQ index**.

All theories, hypotheses, conjectures, and conclusions are based on scientific studies and on the collective wisdom of the greatest minds and spiritual leaders known to human history. With science as our justification, and using logic and deductive reasoning, we will explore all aspects of a whole life, fulfilled and worth-living. The scientific method is the best way, since our species must attempt to find the truth about every and any aspect of life. It does have some limitations, as our current state of knowledge is only a fraction of the overall wisdom available to all living creatures. However, the scientific method offers methodical, repeatable, predictable, and testable procedures for the outcomes of all hypotheses. It is the most certain way we currently have to get to the truth of theories.

> *The good thing about science is that It is true whether or not*
>
> *you believe in it.*
>
> — Neil deGrasse Tyson.

With the application of the scientific process and the combined wisdom of our forefathers and trailblazers, we will investigate our evolution, our current state of overall health, fitness, and joy. We will explore ways to let go of the current vices and sufferings that are preventing us from achieving enlightenment, holistic fitness, and happiness.

PROLOGUE

Believe nothing, no matter where you read it or who

said it, no matter if I have said it, unless it agrees with your

own reason and your own common sense.

— Buddha

Four million years ago, as a response to changing environmental conditions, the evolution of human bipedalism — from quadrupedal primates — began with one single step. From that day onward, a cascade of constant adaptations would ultimately culminate in the complex biomechanical human body we all possess. One brave primate — or maybe a very hungry one — decided to get out of the comfort of the jungle canopies and move into the high grasses of the open savanna. As she moved into the open abyss, her body was trembling, and her instincts were yelling to be in constant vigilance for predators. To see her way out of the tall grasses and find a path forward, she awkwardly stood on just two legs — not a small feat for a quadruped. After several trials, she stumbled and eventually managed several steps in her newly erect position. Her body — not used to this position — ached and quickly commanded her to go back down on her four legs; however, she knew

1

she must persist in moving forward. With unrelenting practice, determination, and thousands of trials and errors, she started to master the task, and her descendants—Homo sapiens—would ultimately manage the art of walking on two legs. Due to this simple step, her descendants—humans—mastered the art of bipedalism, and they embarked on their eternal quest for meaning. This quest would ultimately cause, and paradoxically cure, all of humanity's ills. Seven fundamental truths account for the specific sources and solutions of these human tribulations as well as the creation of happiness: I call these "The Seven Noble Truths."

As Homo sapiens mastered the complex tasks of walking, running, hunting, and gathering, new mechanical and physical stresses started to forge and shape the human body and muscular structures. Evolutionary processes over millions of years played their role to ensure humans were able to successfully survive and thrive. The result was the natural, physically fit human. Her appearance, musculature, and overall body structures—or phenotypes—were all optimized by natural selection to endow her with the best tools to survive, reproduce, and conserve the species. Only the fit had, and continues to have, the opportunity to continue to reproduce; the unfit eventually dies down by way of natural selection, also known as "survival of the fittest."

The most significant evolutionary development of early humans pertained to their brains. The development of the brain—our key competitive advantage over all species—brought with it mental, spiritual, and additional biomechanical stresses that are unique, as far as we know, to humans. At some point during this brain's development, arts, communication, social structures, knowledge-seeking, and spiritual concerns started to appear. These emerged in tandem with all the possibilities that lead to breakdowns and suffering. As humans continued to evolve mentally and to increase their use of tools and accumulation of knowledge, a new concern was born beyond surviving and reproducing. Humanity started the search for meaning and metaphysical truths. Human priorities moved to higher-order levels of concern and worry. The search for happiness, joy, contentment, and fulfillment took center-stage in the human quest. These evolutionary concerns persist today, and the forces driving these changes are the main foundation of *evolutionary fitness*.

Nature provides all wild animals with their optimum levels of fitness, which constantly change to adapt to the prevailing conditions. The human-animal and its brain-derived artificial evolution gave birth to the "unfit human." As civilizations grew and expanded, the primal needs of all humans were being covered by industrialization and mechanical processes. While these innovations made life, food gathering, and surviving easier than ever before, they also birthed much of the disease, suffering, and unfit lifestyle of the modern human.

Charles Darwin, a brilliant scientist of the nineteenth century, revolutionized science, in concert with other scientists, with his theory of evolution. In 1859, he published his famous book, *On the Origin of Species*. His scientific discovery is today the unifying theory of the life sciences, explaining all the diversity of life. One of his central ideas is the fact that all life has descended over time from a common ancestor. It is this idea of evolution — and how it relates to fitness and happiness — that we will explore in this book. We will explore the foundation of the human body from a natural, holistic, and spiritual standpoint, and explore the mind-body connection. A healthy link between mind and body is paramount for reaching happiness. If the body ails, then it is impossible for its owner to achieve happiness. Evolutionary forces shape the form and functions of the body. Evolutionary fitness is the understanding of how these forces have transformed our bodies and how they continue to optimize the body for its environment. Understanding these correlations can result in a fit body and a happy existence. The body is the "hardware" part of our whole, while the soul or spiritual aspect of our well-being is the "software". We will look at both hardware and software through a holistic approach, considering all factors relevant to fitness and happiness. Lastly, I will offer a way to measure these factors. The Fitness Quotient — FQ Index — is a relative way to assess one's overall fitness. Efenians are the followers of this holistic, healthy way of life.

Holistic fitness is the optimum state of well-being a human can obtain. One must consider not only the physical aspects of fitness but also the biochemical, environmental, and spiritual aspects. To be "fit" means to be at one's peak of physical, mental, and spiritual performance. Happiness is a state of joy; it is a requirement of holistic fitness. After all primordial and social needs are met, balance is achieved, and the highest state of internal peace is reached, one gets closer to being holistically fit and happy. The holistic approach looks at the body as self-healing and self-regulating—a perfectly tuned machine. Nature, over millions of years of evolution, has continually changed the definition of a fit body by creating mutations, adaptations, and endless conditions of trial and error. Only those conditions that provide competitive advantages and help organisms continue to thrive and reproduce are maintained. This balance creates the self-healing and self-regulating mechanisms of all organisms, and these mechanisms, operating at their optimum potential, create the fit organism.

With these considerations of holistic health and happiness in mind, we will talk about ways to measure your overall fitness level, and I will provide you with tools to obtain your maximum level of fitness. We will consider all levels of fitness as we survey the available paths. Consider a hypothetical top athlete in peak physical shape. Most measures of physical fitness will declare her to be a fit human. But if this athlete's stress level causes her to consider suicide or performance-enhancing drugs she takes cause long-term damage; I would conclude she is not a "fit" athlete. Her physical-rating markers may be high, but her chemical, emotional, and spiritual indexes are exceptionally low. To be optimally fit, she must successfully address all relevant sources of ills; only then will she find happiness and holistic fitness. Holistic health is the overall approach to fitness we will explore.

Efenians commit to total mental and physical health. To be Efenian is a way of living. I will show you how to become an Efenian and why this is the only path to holistic health and happiness. This lifestyle takes into consideration all aspects of physical and mental fitness; it offers a complete way to look at all facets of a life worth living. "Fitness" in this context refers to the total health of body and mind. To be considered an

PROLOGUE

Efenian, one must follow Efenian principles and achieve an FQ of ninety or higher. Efenians are not members or followers of a cult, religion, diet, or any type of club; to be Efenian is simply to maintain a way of life,

making a commitment to be the best you can be with the ideal form and expression of your inner self reflected in your interactions with the world. We will review how to adopt this way of life.

A glance back in history shows us the Spartans, formidable warriors in ancient Greece (431-404 B.C), known for their outstanding physical abilities and fighting skills. Spartan culture was centered on loyalty to the state and military service. At the early age of seven, boys were socialized in a state-sponsored military education known as "Agoge". This system emphasized duty, discipline, and endurance. The Spartans' lifestyle helped them achieve the highest level of *physical fitness* but not necessarily *mental fitness*. Athenians, on the other hand, were more dedicated to the pursuit of knowledge and development of the mind. Their society gave birth to one of the greatest philosophers of all time: Socrates. Socrates is credited as one of the founders of Western philosophy. The Efenians' way of life creates individuals possessing elements from both cultures: physical fitness and mental fitness. We will explore these two in detail in the upcoming chapters. This book is about scientific arguments as to why the Efenians' way of life is the only way of life. The Efenian's way promotes proper nutrition, exercise, strengthening the body, feeding and calming the mind, meditation, and increasing happiness. When one dedicates one's life to the pursuit of happiness and overall fitness, the benefits are many and clearly visible. By adopting the Efenian's way, you will obtain:

1. A lean, muscular, and healthy body
2. Abundant energy and vitality
3. Clarity of mind (top-performing brain functions)
4. Age delaying
5. Better quality of life (heightened contentment level)
6. Increased laughter and enjoyment

7. A robust immune system (resistant to diseases)
8. A positive outlook on life (reduced and minimized stresses)
9. Wisdom and understanding (lifelong learning)
10. A happier life overall

Let us start our journey.

Stardust

Out of a temple, a young monk emerges,

Fetching for answers, we've been pondering for ages.

'To thy mountain peak must head,' life's trek!

Oh, God's food, dare not neglect.

'Let's go now, down,' thy paths be found

Many tools abound; take me to the ground.

My end is near, no fear, found destiny light

Many fires as one shine bright!

—The Efenian

PART ONE: The First Noble Truth

The Body is Thy Temple

We must, however, acknowledge, as it seems to me, that man

with all his noble qualities...still bears in his bodily frame

the indelible stamp of his lowly origin.

—Charles Darwin

A house for the entirety of the self must be perfect in its construction, flawless in its adaptation, and ideal in its connection to our soul — that is our body. We take our bodies for granted, believing that they will last us forever and serve us well despite our abuses, mistreatments, and neglects. However, that is an illusion. The body is not only finite but breaks down often, especially when neglected. A person who asserts the body is important, yet their actions speak otherwise, is not being truthful to themselves. To firmly state that, "Yes, my body is my temple," an individual must follow this affirmation with the purposeful action that maintains, grows, nurtures, and ultimately, reveres the temple that is the body.

Charles Robert Darwin—creator of the theory of evolution—described the body forms, phenotypes, of hundreds of species and gave science the reasons why such characteristics came about. Darwin first shocked the religious Victorian society of the 19th century by suggesting that animals and humans shared a common ancestry. His science-based biology appealed to the rising class of professional scientists and, by the time of his death, his concepts had spread across all of science, politics, and literature. In order to understand bodies and their evolutionary functions, Darwin is our best ambassador.

⬤

Charles Darwin was born in 1809 in Shropshire, England. He was the fifth of six children of Robert Darwin—a wealthy doctor—and Susannah Darwin. Both of his grandfathers, Erasmus Darwin and Josiah Wedgwood, were abolitionists. Both of his parents were Unitarian—a Christian movement that believes that God is one person, as opposed to the Holy Trinity of most Christian denominations. By the time he was eight years old, young Darwin had already developed a taste for natural history and collecting items. His mother died during this time; after that, he was cared for by his three elder sisters. He enrolled with his brother Erasmus at the nearby Anglican Shrewsbury boarding school. His overbearing father, an astute medical observer, taught him much about psychology. Darwin hated studying the Classics at the traditional Anglican Shrewsbury school. Science in public schools during this time was considered dehumanizing and, for his work in chemistry, he was condemned by his headmaster and nickname "Gas" by his schoolmates.

His father, concerned with 16-year-old Darwin only being interested in game shooting, sent him to study medicine at Edinburgh University in 1825. Darwin would later reflect that he learned almost nothing during this his two years at Edinburgh and stated that it was mostly a formative experience—even though that was the best science education of the times. At school, he learned chemistry, geology, and plant classification. He spent the summer of 1825 as an apprentice doctor, helping his father treat the poor of Shropshire, before going to the University of Edinburgh Medical School which, at the time, was considered to be the best medical school in the United Kingdom. He found the lectures dull and surgery distressing, so he frequently neglected his studies. His neglect of medical studies annoyed his father so much that he sent him to Christ's College, Cambridge, to study for a Bachelor of Arts.

By 1828, Darwin was pursuing his interest in collecting beetles. Some of his findings were published in James Francis Stephen's *Illustrations of British Entomology*. He became a close friend and follower of botany professor John Stevens Henslow and met other leading naturalists who saw scientific work as religious natural theology. Darwin stayed at Cambridge until June 1831. He studied Paley's *Natural Theology or Evidence of the Existence and Attributes of the Deity*, which argues for divine design in nature, explaining adaptation as God acting through laws of nature. After leaving Sedgwick in Wales, Darwin returned home to find a letter from Henslow proposing him as a suitable naturalist for a self-funded supernumerary place on HMS Beagle with Captain Robert Fitzroy. The ship was to depart in four weeks on an expedition to chart the coastline of South America. The voyage lasted almost five years. He spent most of that time investigating geology and making natural history collections. He kept careful notes of his observations and theoretical speculations. His specimens were sent to Cambridge, together with letters and copies of his journals. During one of these voyages, Darwin made a major find of a fossil bone in the south of Patagonia. The fossil, which was of a large, extinct mammal, was next to modern seashells, which indicated recent extinction with no sign of change in climate or catastrophe. He identified the little-known Megatherium by a tooth and its association with bony armour, which had at first seemed to him like a giant version of the armour of local armadillos.

By 1837, after his return to England, Darwin was postulating in his red notebook about the possibility that "one species does change into another," to explain the geographical distribution of living species, such as the rheas, and of extinct ones, such as the strange extinct mammal, Macrauchenia, which resembled a giant guanaco, a llama relative. His thoughts on lifespan, on asexual reproduction, on sexual reproduction, and on the variation in offspring, were that these are "to adapt and alter the race to changing world" — thus explaining the Galapagos tortoises, mockingbirds, and rheas. He sketched branching descent in which "it is absurd to talk of one animal being higher than another," thereby discarding Jean Baptiste Lamarck's independent lineages progressing to higher forms — Lamarck was also a great scientist of the times working on evolution theories. Darwin created his bold theory in private, and it was not until decades later that he finally gave it full public view, in *On the Origin of Species (1859)*, a book that changed the course of Western society and thought.

On April 19, 1882, Darwin suffered from angina, had a seizure, and died of a heart attack. His last words to his wife were, "I am not the least afraid of death — Remember what a good wife you have been to me — tell all my children to remember how good they have been to me."

Darwin is considered the father of evolution. Although he did not have any knowledge of genetics, he was able to make conclusive arguments as to why and how species develop and evolve over time. His two main points were that diverse groups of animals evolved from one or a few common ancestors, and that the mechanism by which this evolution takes place is natural selection.

CHAPTER 1: LET THERE BE LIGHT

INFINITY — A MOMENT IN TIME

To keep the body in good health is a duty... Otherwise, we

shall not be able to keep our mind strong.

— Buddha

"*A*nd then there was light"... 13.7 billion years ago, the origin of the universe, the genesis of the entire human race, began with a huge bang, known in science as the Big Bang Theory. After, millions and millions of years of trial and error, countless optimizations, natural selection, and Darwinian evolution, we arrived at an optimum-adapted Homo sapiens genus — the human species — possessing a uniquely developed brain, superiorly evolved body, and unsurpassed intelligence, enough to advance her to the top of the food chain. That is how we all began our existence. Since the production of the very first elementary particles, atoms, elements and, eventually, molecules and microorganisms, the natural evolutionary forces have been shaping the destination of our current human form and function based on the prevailing environment, current conditions, competition, and need to survive and procreate. Evolution has been painting our canvas of life through our entire historical time. We, as a human race, appear to be the winners of the evolutionary lottery. However, despite this seemingly lucky development, and after thousands of years of civilization, we stand today as one of the sickest and fragile species on our planet.

Our entire existence is in a very delicate and thin balance, with a very narrow set of conditions perfectly adapted to life—we call this the Goldilocks condition: not too hot, not too cold, simply perfect. Today, humanity is in a precarious situation. There is a trend of ever-increasing chronic diseases, obesity, mental illness, and overall unhealthy and poorly functional bodies and minds. The average life expectancy has steadily increased worldwide during the last few decades; however, the number of new diseases and syndromes continue to climb, despite our technology and medical advances. In the United States, there is currently an epidemic of obesity. Chronic diseases and conditions such as heart diseases, strokes, cancers, type 2 diabetes, obesity, and dementia are among the most common, costly, and preventable of all health problems. According to the World Health Organization (WHO), chronic diseases will soon account for almost three-quarters of all deaths worldwide. Even with the continued increase in life expectancy, the decrease of child mortality, and the improvement of emergency and critical care, the quality of overall fitness for most individuals have decreased.

Our modern societies, with their ever-increasing pace of living, higher stress levels, exposure to synthetic chemicals, overconsumption of calories, and nutrient-poor, calorie-rich foods are now mostly artificially modified environments that are making us sicker every day. This new industrial environment and the forces associated with it are accelerating changes in our bodies that nature did not intend. This form of artificial evolution is one of the main causes of today's increase in diseases and lower overall fitness. Natural evolution is a slow process, and nature likes to take its time to produce radical changes in our DNA and phenotypes. The mechanism of natural selection is ultimately responsible for our total fitness and overall health. It is important to understand how these mechanisms are working, how they are affecting our bodies and minds, and how one can give one's self the best chance to continue to evolve in the best possible way, to compete and survive in our chosen living environment. We need to consider all the factors affecting this evolution: this is a holistic approach. Holistic includes not only the factors contained in nature and the environment but also all the nurture factors, as well. Nature and nurture work in concert to produce our bodily and mental states. Nature, in this argument, is referring to the natural changes the body goes through as a result of evolution, while nurture is more of the body changes due to artificially human-generated environments. This is sometimes referred to as epigenetics changes or changes beyond the gene itself. A trait inherited from the parents is an example of a nature-derived change, while a genetic change — let us say, due to exposure to a carcinogenic substance which turns certain genes on — is an example of nurture.

Bodies forged under evolutionary fitness

An understanding of the theory of evolution is paramount to understanding the human body: its origin, its concerns, and its past and future. Understanding how our bodies have evolved helps us see more clearly where the ever-evolving body may be going. Deep knowledge of the origin of our bodies gives us the tool needed to better take care of them and to seek proactive ways to make them function at their best. Charles Darwin's theory of evolution states[6] that evolution happens by natural selection. The theory of evolution is based on the idea that all species are related, coming from a common ancestor, and they gradually change over time to adapt to the prevailing environmental conditions. This theory is our best explanation of the current evolutionary path of our human body. One mechanism of this theory is genetic variation. Genetic variation in the population affects the physical characteristics (phenotype) of the species. The variation is due to differences in the genes. These variations, in turn, may give one

14

individual advantages over others, and may dictate the success of the species overall. Evolution, in biology, is the change in the characteristics of a species over several generations, and it relies on the process of natural selection. The species with the best-suited characteristics are more likely to thrive, find food, avoid predation, resist disease, and ultimately be better at surviving and reproducing. This is a competitive advantage that allows them to continue to propagate. Those individuals that are poorly adapted to their environment are less likely to reproduce, and their genes will not be passed to future generations. The process of natural selection ensures that those species with the best characteristics are the ones that continue to reproduce and pass along their competitive advantages to their offspring. This mechanism plays an important role in the current state of humanity.

One classic example of the theory of natural selection is the evolution of the Peppered Moth, in the mid-1700s in England, just before the onset of the industrial revolution. The Peppered Moths had a pale whitish color on their wings, with black spots. This coloring scheme allowed them to avoid predation by blending with the pale-colored bark of the tree in their environment. As the industrial revolution rolled on, pollution-filled stacks covered the trees, buildings, and the overall environment where the moths were living. As a result, the moths with the lighter color became extremely easy to spot by predators (birds), as they were not able to blend in with the bark as before. A few moths of a darker color were able to better camouflage with the now soot-stained trees, and therefore they acquired a competitive advantage over the lighter moth. Over time, this change in the environment led to the darker moths becoming more common and the pale moths rarer. This is a classic evolution at work. The human body evolved using this same process of natural selection. Our post-industrial way of living, which includes food that is genetically modified food (GMO), is filled with hormones, treated with high quantities of antibiotics, highly processed (and devoid of nutrients), and chock full of refined sugars and salt, is causing genetic changes in our bodies which are the main causes of the deterioration of overall fitness and the increasing prevalence of chronic diseases. Genetics can today explain in detail how these changes are being performed, preserved, and passed on to future generations. Our genes contain all our evolutionary histories. We look as we do because of all the genetic changes that affected our ancestors.

Evolution is constantly changing our bodies. By being aware of "artificial evolution," we can begin to understand the function and form of the body, and we can then proceed to act wisely, choosing to do things like eating the proper nutrition, avoiding being exposed to dangerous chemicals and environments, and reducing excessive levels of stress, factors that can lead to negative traits and phenotypes. All these factors lead to the breakdown of our body and, through gene expressions (epigenetic), they turn on genes that can harm us and lead us into unhealthy paths. Considering evolutionary fitness also gets us closer to living a natural life, as nature is the correct way to evolve (slowly, purposefully, and with a relentless aim to optimize the body). Nature – a more natural way of living – is the best chance for optimal health and happiness. Changes in DNA and epigenetic are the basic units of inheritance. These changes, whether beneficial or not, are passed onto future generations. Natural selection in humans is being substituted by *artificial selection,* as we continue to choose profits over natural health. Artificial evolution is a product of the powerful corporations and special interest groups that have as their primary goal the mandate to increase shareholder value (i.e., maximize profit). This happens when we create artificial products (like highly processed food, antibiotics, neurotoxins, carcinogens, and other dangerous chemically synthesized products), and we drastically and irresponsibly change the environment in which we live. The body responds to toxic exposures – mostly from artificial, human-made products – by turning on some genes and causing diseases of the bodies.

Body—A self-healing, self-regulating sublimity

In nature, biological fitness—also known as Darwinian fitness—is the ability to survive to reproductive age, find a mate, and produce offspring. The more offspring an organism produces during its lifetime, the greater its biological fitness. Our definition of fitness is much broader in the sense that it is not only biological but mental as well. Our brain cortex evolved to give us a unique and superior advantage over all species on Earth. Fitness, in our context, is the ability to successfully reproduce while having an optimum state of joy. Biology plays a particularly important role in the function of our bodies. The mind/body connection keeps these two interlinked, and only when these are in harmony can we claim a true state of fitness. The body is a perfectly tuned machine: it self-regulates and self-heals. Given that we provide it the proper nutrients and mental environment, the body creates a very strong defense system—the immune system—which keeps the body in an optimum healthy state and, when attacked by a pathogen, it kills all the foreign substances and brings the body back to health. This concept is overly critical to a healthy style of living.

An Efenian style of living will recognize this fact as key to living the best possible life. If we honestly believe that the body is self-healing and self-regulating, we then will not be second-guessing our nature and trying to alter our physiology with man-made chemicals—especially when we are not sure of the true root cause of the diseases. In our heavily medicated society, a person who becomes sick is very prone to take antibiotics for simple allergies and infections that, if left alone, the body would eliminate on its own, thus becoming stronger in the process. Additionally, if the body is left alone to fight the infection, it will develop immunity to the pathogen and fend off any future attack by the same enemy. Individuals ought to give the body the time to heal itself, as long as there is not an emergency or a situation that demands immediate intervention. I am not against the use of medicine or medical procedures. In a time of emergencies, these procedures and medication can be lifesaving. However, I am advocating moderation and giving the body enough time to heal itself whenever appropriate.

The standard care in the United States is done primarily by the MD – Doctor of Medicine. These doctors are educated and certified and work with a philosophy of the allopathic model. The allopathic models refer to a system in which medical doctors and other practitioners treat symptoms and diseases using drugs, radiation, or surgery – also called biomedicine and Western medicine. They cover the maintenance of health, including both acute care and prevention. A growing trend in the medical industry is the DO – Doctor of Osteopathic Medicine. These DO doctors have a completely different approach to practicing medicine, as their philosophy involves treating the mind, the body, and the spirit. It is a more holistic approach. When one realizes that the body is self-healing and self-regulating, then the DO approach is a much more sensible one to medicine and health. And rather than looking at just the symptoms, as MD doctors do, the DO doctors seek to treat the root cause of the diseases. The American Osteopathic Association (AOA) says the key is that osteopathic medicine treats the "whole person." This new wave of doctor is looking at the whole body and finding ways to cure the real cause of the ills, not just the symptoms, as well as treating the whole body and mind, with minimal usage of artificial drugs and procedures. This is an especially important trend in medicine but, unfortunately, according to the Federation of State Medical Boards (FSMB), in 2012, nine out of ten practicing doctors in the US were MDs or allopathic physicians. The body is a very fine-tuned machine, with a super-powerful computer (brain) that, when given the proper nutrition, care, and time to heal, will do so. We should not run to the hospital on the first sign of the disease – unless it is a medical emergency or chronic condition. We should first give the body a chance to fight the maladies and, by doing so, the body will make itself stronger and develop resistance to the disease and others like it. Other instances in which we do not allow the body to become stronger is when we over-clean, wash our hands way too much, worry about any exposure to pathogens, and are in general paranoid about any exposure to dirt and microbes. By exposing the body to natural dirt and some unclean conditions, one is giving the body an opportunity to fight many types of pathogens and, by this process, training the internal army – the immune system – to be ready for all types of intruders. The immune system is then becoming stronger and expanding its arsenals of pathogen-fighting weapons. A strong immune system is the hallmark of a fit individual.

The MD approach of the medical industry today is to consider an individual to be healthy if the individual's key parameters are within a certain prescribed value range. (for example, blood pressure of 120/80 mmHg, sugar levels of less than 100 mg/dL, etc.). This is known as the homeostasis approach. The main issue with this approach is that the individual can have all her parameters within the prescribed value and still be on the road to major chronic diseases. Consider the example of an individual who is, according to all the lab measurements, "healthy." Her cholesterol, blood pressure, sugar, triglycerides, and all other key parameters are within her recommended range. However, she is living a very unhealthy life— eating fast food, having mental stress at work, and living a "toxic" life that has not caught up with the individual yet. The homeostatic approach will not be able to help this individual— since her parameters do not as yet show the breakdown—and she is on the road to a major crash. The homeostasis approach is not proactive or preventive. It only addresses the "current" state of the individual. An alternative approach that is much more efficient than this homeostasis model is to consider all the factors that control the overall health of the individual. When it comes to being treated for an illness, if you do not need to go to a hospital, it is to one's benefit to look for a Doctor of Osteopathic Medicine. These types of doctors will give the best care possible, as they are looking at the whole body, not just symptoms.

A classic Indian parable, *The Blind Men and an Elephant*, tells the story of six blind sojourners that come across different parts of an elephant in their journey. The group of blind men heard that a strange animal, called an elephant, had been brought to town, but none of them were aware of its shape and form. Out of curiosity, they said: "We must inspect and know it by touch, of which we are capable." They sought it, and when they found it, they set out to inspect it. The first person, who landed on the trunk, said: "This being is like a thick snake." For another one whose hand reached its ear, it seemed to be a kind of fan. Another person, whose hand was upon its leg, said, "The elephant is a pillar, like a tree-trunk." The blind man who placed his hands upon the side said the elephant "is a wall." Another who felt its tail described it as a rope. The last felt its tusk, stating, "The elephant is that which is hard, smooth, and like a spear."

The moral of this parable is that humans tend to claim absolute truth based on their limited, subjective experience, as they ignore other people's limited, subjective experience which may be equally true. It is also a great demonstration of what happens when we only consider some parts and not the whole. When traditional MDs just look at your stomach pain, for example, and do not consider your current state of mind, they are practicing just looking at the leg of the elephant. This beautiful analogy reminds us to be vigilant when trying to uncover the truth, and to be open to other points of view, always looking at the whole instead of just its parts.

The Efenian way of life entails looking at the individual as a whole collection of systems that all interconnect and work very closely with each other. These networks are finely tuned and must be treated as such. Since the body is self-regulating, it would be futile to look at trying to optimize your overall health by just looking at a few factors. If one hopes to be holistic, then one must look at all factors affecting body fitness. The parameters of optimum fitness to be considered are the physical body (muscle structure), the current state of physical stress (any pains or current illnesses), the chemical stress to which your body is being exposed, the type of food you eat (diets), your mental health (mind), your breathing health, and your overall body's ability to perform work and resist stress (energy). We will look at all these factors and show you how they relate to your overall health and fitness.

There is nothing either good or bad, but thinking makes it so.

—William Shakespeare, Hamlet

Happiness—The Body and Mind as One

The founding fathers of the United States of America, during the writing of the Declaration of Independence, added a statement on the constitution declaring that, "We hold these truths to be self-evident, that all men are created equal, that they are endowed by their Creator with certain unalienable rights, that among these are life, liberty and the pursuit of happiness." They considered the pursuit of happiness to be a basic right of human endeavor. One can easily agree that searching for happiness is our ultimate goal. However, most people cannot agree on exactly what it means to be happy. Widely accepted is that happiness is associated with a high level of economic status, the search for monetary and material wealth. The more material things that one has, the happier that person is considered to be. These views are ill-conceived and are too narrow to truly consider the full spectrum of being happy. Being happy is a requirement of being fit. If one is unhappy, then the body becomes ill in response to the unhappy input and the stress put on it. One cannot happen without the other.

A child's birth is analogous to the creation of the universe. With a big bang or a big push in the case of a child, life is thrust upon existence. Most people recognize life when they see it. We can tell whether something is alive or dead. Characteristic of life includes the ability to self-replicate, have motion, exhibit growth and decay, among others. However, biologists and philosophers cannot agree on a simple definition. Life is too complex—even more when we add consciousness to it—so when it comes to life, we can only refer to the *"state of being alive."* As we look at the state of optimum fitness, we will consider the fact we are programmed with a prime objective: "preserve life and propagate the species." To this end and considering that humans are at the top of the food chain, we have expanded our prime directive and added a general principle of "search for happiness." It is not enough to just be fit or to be able to preserve and multiply the species; we also have the need to be happy. It is to this later pursuit that we will look in order to search for a holistic approach to overall fitness.

A complete description of happiness will include freedom for these four basic tenets:

1. Body Freedom: Consider a body that is in optimum physical shape, has a strong immune system, and quickly responds to any illness or temporary attack from any foreign pathogens. This body will be an optimized body. A body that is not in optimum fitness (weak immune systems, low-to-no muscular structure) will be easily ill and will not be free from bodily breakdown.

2. Mind Freedom: This refers to being free of the negative thoughts and restriction that the mind puts on the body and that lead to diseases and ills. Being mentally free means always being in a state of peaceful bliss and positive energy, or at least most of the time. A state of depression or a state of mental stress will produce physical stress and eventually ills on the body. This is what I refer to as mind freedom or mind mastery — a mind that is at peace knows how to handle stress and is in harmonious balance with the body.

3. Material Freedom: Suffering stems from our desires. Desiring material things and possessions can lead to suffering. Even when we obtain these material things, we still yearn for more. This vicious circle of desire leads to suffering, mental stress, and eventually ills of the body. Material freedom refers to being able to let go of material desires. This is a very mature trait and can only be obtained after many years of wisdom and reflection, questioning the nature of the profoundly important aspects of life.

4. Financial Freedom: The model of the prevailing social system of modern countries includes being able to take care of all your basic needs — shelter, food, security, etc. — by yourself. In order to be able to address these concerns, one will need a minimum of monetary currency where work is no longer necessary. This amount of money is what I call your specific financial freedom amount. This will be different for different people. An average of four to five million dollars on today's current USD monetary value seems to be around the right amount to afford financial freedom, assuming a steady cash flow of passive income.

Because fitness and happiness are so eternally coupled, one needs to address all freedoms above before we can obtain holistic health and happiness. We will address all these in terms of the mental aspect of fitness in future chapters. The best body is within — we just need to bring it out.

CHAPTER 2: HOMO SAPIENS

BODY—THE TEMPLE OF THE SOUL

Without health, life is not life; it is only a state of languor and suffering - an image of death.

— Buddha

T he evolution of our current bodies is like the birth of a new river. The river does not decide what course it will end up on; the path of least resistance ultimately defines the final winding banks that the river will inherit. As our ancestors came out of the oceans and moved through the evolutionary branches of the tree of life, we evolved into our present phenotype. Homo sapiens morphed into having the bodies we have inherited on the evolutionary lottery of life. We evolved to have legs, hands, eyes, ears, backbone, and a myriad of perfectly adapted cells and organs. Like the river, the human body was the result of our environment and the reaction to all the force that acted on it, as well. The function of

24

the human body was to be the vessel of all our actions and reactions to the universe. As such, individuals cannot exist without some form of a body. Nature and evolutionary fitness provided the optimum physical structure for the body, given our environment and living situation. This is important because, without a body, as far as we know today, one will not survive or successfully multiply the species. This is what allows all other species to continue to evolve and reproduce. A functional body is a primal necessity to carnal existence.

Currently, artificial human evolution is accelerating and reshaping our bodies in ways that are not beneficial in the long term. The obesity epidemic in the US is a great example of the current artificial evolution that we are living today, and it is producing unprecedented levels of unfitness and many sick individuals. If we return to our natural state of health and fitness, we will optimize our fitness. The body is a temple: one needs to treat it as such. A temple must be maintained with the utmost care, be kept meticulously clean, organized, neat, and only have the most basic needs fulfilled to ensure proper function. This is a great analogy, and it is the type of treatment that the body requires if the individual is to have optimal health.

The connection between the body and the soul we call our consciousness. It is near impossible to separate the body and soul as these two make the whole which is ourselves. This chapter will focus primarily on the physical aspect that is our body and will consider the mind, and the mind-body connection, in later chapters.

Take care of the body, and the body will take care of you.

—JC Paulino

The body is your temple—care for it

The body is the temple of your soul. It is perfectly attuned with your mind, and they both work on a harmonious symphony. When one's body suffers, the mind suffers; when the body ails, the mind ails. This duality can only exist harmoniously if both parts are working optimally and together. A healthy mind can only exist in a healthy body. The body and mind connection are one of the most mysterious things, and science has not been able to fully explain it. We conjecture about consciousness, and most scientists agree that consciousness is real, but we quickly get in trouble when we try to define it and explain its true nature.

There is an abundance of theories of consciousness, from metaphysical to quantum theory, and not all agreeing on their hypothesis; however, most people would agree that a body in optimum shape is the cornerstone to a fit and healthy body. When considering the duality of the body and soul, one cannot exist in full harmony and health – fitness – without the other. It is for this reason that we must take care of the body to ensure that we can keep the harmonious link between body and soul. A "sick" body, or a body that is not optimum, is not the proper vessel for a holistically fit person. We abuse the body when we expose it to toxins, junk foods, alcohols, and non-nutritious substances, and when we do not exercise or do physical activities to help the body heal. We only get one body in our life cycle, so we must treat our bodies as such – a precious commodity. Let us assume that an individual possesses the most precious vehicle ever created. He would take impeccable care of it by keeping it safe, clean, and in optimum shape. This individual would give this possession the utmost care and maintenance. Why, then, could he not do the same for his body?

If one honestly believes that the body is the temple of the soul, then one must do all that is necessary to keep it in optimal shape, devoid of excessive fats, with abundant muscular structures, and in a maximum healthy state. To keep the body fit, one must give it proper nutrition, not provide it with sub-optimal fuel (processed food), hazardous chemicals or drugs (artificial chemicals, harsh cleaners, cosmetics, fluoridated water, iodized salt, etc.). Exposure and consumption of synthetic chemicals produces chemical stress in the body which could result in severe or chronic diseases. As residents of modern society, this is a risk we face daily. The government, the chemical industries, the medical industry, and all other consumer industries have their own agenda in mind, and it is not necessarily your health. Educated consumers need to be vigilant, well informed, and ultimately be able to compare different points of view and make their own science-based decision with the available facts. Thankfully, we live today in an information age where data is readily available; however, the individual must still be capable of reading through mounds of fine print and come up with the best-informed decision on any potentially damaging, toxic exposures. Individuals need to consider all points of view when deciding on what is best for the body and use all available evidence to arrive at the optimal solution.

For instance, the white coat syndrome is when we just believe what a person is saying because they are wearing a "white coat". The person surrenders her reason and gives credibility in totality to the person on the other side — who is supposedly the expert. The issue with the white coat syndrome is that doctors — as well as many other professionals — are often wrong. As a matter of fact, doctors kill more people than car accidents. A recent report from Johns Hopkins's study claims that more than 250,000 people in the United States die each year from medical errors (other reports claim the number to be as high as 440,000). So, when it comes to your body, research, second opinions, and methodical and logical analysis are the only roads to take if one hopes to find the truth. Taking care of the body entails being a steward of it, carefully studying any and all substances that are going into our body (i.e., their effects). One needs to be vigilant, by not only looking at the consumption of chemical substances by mouth, but at any type of exposure, like radiation, skin exposure, heat, and over-stimulating visual inputs. We gather information by using our five senses; we must be aware of the effects of all these inputs on body health.

Consider the skin, the largest organ of the body. We are constantly being exposed to harsh fragrances, creams, UV rays, and many other chemicals that are potentially hazardous to the skin. What is the effect of

27

these chemicals on the fitness level? The chemical, pharmaceutical, food, and water industries all expose the body to hundreds of thousands of synthetic chemicals, the effects of which have not been determined — especially when these are used in combination for long periods of time. The level of exposure, furthermore, needs to be considered in terms of all senses. A foul smell can be as deadly and as toxic as food or a very loud sound. All sensory information carries with it a level of risks when the exposure is too high or toxic.

⚬⚮⚬

Body fitness is much more than just physical appearance or sexual attraction. The body functions are many, and all are intimately connected to the mind, without which there would not be the self. Without a fit body, one cannot obtain happiness. Here is a thought experiment: consider the last time you felt lousy, or when you had a cold or a minor disease — how did you feel mentally? It is highly likely you felt tired, energy-deprived, lethargic, and overall miserable. No state of joy exists without holistic health. The personal temple is one's most valued asset. A full understanding of this concept implies that the person will never abuse the body. Body misfortunes and abuses can take many forms and sometimes the individual may not even be conscious of them. Important factors include proper sleeping — is the individual getting enough rest and meditation? Is the person getting at least 20 minutes of natural sunlight, in order to absorb Vitamin D? Is the person eating organic and plant-based products? Is the individual under a regimen of daily medications or OTC, which have many side effects? We will look at each of these factors individually, but I want you to start thinking about the true meaning of "taking care of your body." Many individuals will claim, "Yes, I am taking care of my body," but when their daily habits are closely monitored, we find all the above breakdowns. The body is the main component of the mind-body connection. A prerequisite to happiness is achieving a fit and healthy body and providing the right conditions for optimum mind-body connections. The body is the vessel of all our actions. The concept of the fit body should also span throughout your whole life cycle — from infancy to the later years. Most people only focus on their young years (ages 18 to 33) to maintain a great body physique — this is less than six percent of the average life!

To holistically evaluate the body on all levels — the physical and the mental — and to accurately measure these, I have created a fitness rating factor named the Fitness Quotient (FQ). FQ is a way to access the overall fitness of the body, considering all important parameters that affect overall health.

The Fitness Quotient (FQ)—Ultimate holistic health metric

The FQ index is a relative number that gives you an overall indication of fitness and well-being. It should be considered as a guideline only, as it is exceedingly difficult to accurately measure overall fitness. One must consider the interactions of all parameters, as well. Using a single number to try to capture the whole fitness state is like using the Dow Jones Index to gauge the whole US economy. Although the DOW Jones is a good indicator of economic activity, it is not a predictor of current or future economic trends. The FQ index should be used in a similar way. It provides a scale value and level that indicates your "relative" fitness level. Once you calculate your FQ value, you can see areas where you are deficient, and consequently, you can take appropriate action to correct the deficiencies. A high FQ value is correlated to overall high happiness and health. If you have an FQ factor of 90 or better, then it is highly likely you are doing all the right things to live the best life you can possibly can, including being in your best physical and mental condition, and in your highest state of happiness.

Fifteen key performance indicators are included in the FQ index. This is a holistic approach in that it considers not only your physical condition, but your emotional state, your biochemical balance, and your happy state. The body is an overly complex and perfectly optimized machine. Nature, using the process of evolution and natural selection, maximizes the fitness level based on the environment and the pressures

29

that it endures. When a balanced state is reached by reducing or eliminating all stresses—physical, chemical, and mental—a state of happiness is accomplished. We will explore these stresses further in subsequent chapters.

The FQ index scale is summarized in Appendix A. Take the test summarized in this appendix, and you will have an overall idea of your fitness level. (You can also evaluate your factor at *Efenians.com*. The scale of the FQ index is from 0 to 100. The test has several areas that are subjective. You will need to be truthful and honest in your response to ensure you get an accurate scale reading. This score is only for your personal use, so there is no sense in either omitting or exaggerating any answers on the test. In a holistic approach, one needs to consider the physical, mental, environmental, chemical, spiritual, and metaphysical aspects of our lives. We value "the pursuit of happiness" as one of the key human rights. The pursuit of this happiness is dependent on obtaining a holistically acceptable level of fitness. When we address all these factors, then we can conclude that we have given ourselves the best chance at happiness. A breakdown or lack of any of these factors will inhibit and or restrict our level of happiness.

The components of the FQ index are broken down into five key categories. These include all major factors of holistic fitness. A high FQ index is also an indicator of joy or happiness. The premise used for this factor is that the body is part of a whole biological system, and in order to be optimally fit, one must be fit physically and mentally.

The Fitness Quotient is one's fitness gauge. All key factors which are relevant to fitness are included in this metric. One key factor that is considered a master factor because, by itself, it can accurately evaluate the physical condition of the individual is the stomach core muscle structures —the "six-pack." This metric is universal as it correlates very strongly with overall fitness. There are very few people who have a six-pack and are not fit. It can also be estimated visually, as one can see the level of definition, size, and symmetric appearance of the six-pack. It is an outstanding metric to use as a general guideline for physical health.

The FQ Index Scale

Level A (Athlete 90-100): This individual has an athletic physique with a proportionally defined muscular structure. A fat percentage of less than 10% (men), 15% (women). No taking of any medications, drugs, or performance enhancers. Mental toughness and a high level of happiness. Most time is spent in a state of flow.

Level B (Above Average 80-89): She has some proportionally defined muscular structure. A fat percentage of less than 15% (men) and 20% (women). No taking of any medications. She is mentally grounded and has relatively high level of happiness.

Level C (Average 70-79): He may show some proportionally defined muscular structure. A fat percentage of less than 20% (men) and 25% (women). One may be taking some medications. Emotionally not completely grounded and relatively mid-level of happiness

Level D (Poor 60-69): She is starting to work on body-muscular structure. A fat percent of higher than 30%. Likely taking medications. Mentally weak and high mood swings. Low level of happiness

Level F (Intervention Needed 0-59): She has one or more critical areas that need immediate attention.

The FQ Components and Concerns

I. *Muscular Composition* (BODY): Body muscle composition and symmetry. It also looks at the composition of fats and overall body stability and mechanical structure:

- *Stomach Type* (Core Muscle Definition). Abs and core muscle structure.
- *Fat percent:* Body fat composition and distribution.
- *Muscular composition:* Overall body muscular definition, size, and structure.

II. Performance Power (BODY): Ability of the body to perform work and flexibility.

- *Flexibility:* Muscle flexibility and ductility.
- *Strength:* Body overall power rating.
- *Stamina:* (Cardio health), speed, and endurance.

III. Chemical Stress (BODY & MIND)

- *Nutrition:* Eating patterns and nutrient profile.
- *Chemical stress:* Chemicals and Medicines exposures directly or indirectly.
- *Environmental stress:* Environmental exposures.

IV. Mental Stress (MIND)

- *Happiness Level:* Current level of mental stress and happiness
- *Mental health state:* Mental illness state. Any onset of actual mental illness.
- *Meditation:* Oxygenation patterns and overall respiratory health. Meditation.

V. Physical Stress State (BODY)

- *Body Illness.* Structural- and nerve-related stresses or illness.
- *Pains and discomforts.* Skeletally- and or structurally induce stress.
- *Body alignment/postures.* Inflammation and miscellaneous body ills.

A fit body—necessity of happiness

The human body comprises many systems, each in charge of specific functions. For instance, the respiratory system is charged with oxygenating all the body cells and removing carbon dioxide and other gaseous toxins from the body. However, no system works in isolation. The body is the holistic harmony of all these systems and is connected via a feedback loop to constantly optimize the body function. When the body is fit, the body systems are taking care of any harmful foreign pathogen quickly and efficiently. A fit body also uses energy efficiently and does not carry any excess fats. It has a muscular level high enough to allow it to do its basic functions at the highest level possible. This optimum level of fitness allows you to focus on the business of improving your overall happiness. One simple definition of happiness is being in a state of joy. If you use this definition, then we can conclude that, if one is sick, in pain and or discomforts—mental or physical, one cannot get to a state of joy. Only when all these stressors are eliminated or reduced to their minimum level can the person start the journey towards a state of joy — obviously, since the body and the mind are intimately connected, they both need to be in optimum shape in order to reach the highest level of happiness.

We will discuss the role of the mind in this equation, but in this chapter, we want to focus on the physical aspect that is the body. Pains of short duration should be viewed as the alarm system of the body. They indicate that there is a specific area that the person needs to take care of it. Pains are a very natural response to the attack of the body, and, without these monitoring signals, the body will not function properly.

We should view pains in a positive light, as they are alerting the body to what we need to correct to get back to the right side of health. Long term pain may require professional assistance — especially chronic and emergency situations. For most pain, one should search for the root cause of the pain, address the deficiency, and give the body the proper nutrients, rest, and meditation so that the body can take care of the pain. The body is a perfectly adapted machine, self-healing, so whenever possible, one should give it the opportunity to perform as such.

Symmetry—fit body causality

A natural body refers to one who is as close to nature as possible, one who avoids consuming artificial products and environments. Although artificial products greatly increase the convenience of modern living, they are created with the idea of maximizing profits for corporations, governments, and shareholders. The use of the products and the benefits to humankind of most products is secondary in nature to the profit equation. Analyze any man-made product in the modern supermarket and you will quickly realize that all of these products are deficient in true nutrients and abundant in sugar and salt, which are the key ingredients that aid in the sale and the overuse of these products. Marketers take advantage of the fact that we love sugar and salt — there is a logical evolutionary reason for this desire as these two products were very scarce at the beginning of industrialization. With the advent of supermarkets and industrialization, however, these two ingredients became superabundant and are the primary ingredients used to sell a cornucopia of synthetic products. A natural body is one who uses sugars in their most natural form — including the especially important fiber component, for example, in fruit form — thereby taking advantage of the millions of years of evolution that went into creating the product. Take honey for example: in natural form, honey is a superfood providing a wealth of mineral-, antioxidant-, carbohydrate-, and cholesterol-balancing properties. A nature-focused body is in balance with his environment and consequently is in the best possible condition of health.

HOMO SAPIENS

Leonardo Davinci's Vitruvian Man celebrates the beauty and proportions of the natural man. It is a mathematically beautiful interpretation of the human body's perfection and its adaptability to the environment. By realizing this evolutionary perfection, we start to appreciate the delicate work of nature in creating the human body. We can all appreciate when a body is symmetrical, muscular, and in good proportion. This natural beauty, captured by Davinci, should be the goal of every human body—not only because of the beauty that such a body possesses, but because of the practical and highly efficient ability that such a body has to function on its environment, to do work, to reproduce, to preserve the species, all of which leads to the state of joy that we refer to as happiness. By sculpturing the body, one pays homage to it.

The response of the body to an outside stimulus is considered a highly intelligent response based on millions of years of evolution. The body is smart about this reaction, and one needs to respect the response of the body and try to understand why it is doing what it is doing. It is for this reason that it is important to have at least a basic understanding of the primary body systems and their functions to be able to take care of the body, and to know when you should leave the body do its magic or when you should seek medical help. This is what being in tune with your body is all about. One should be able to cure most of the common diseases naturally and let the immune system heal the body.

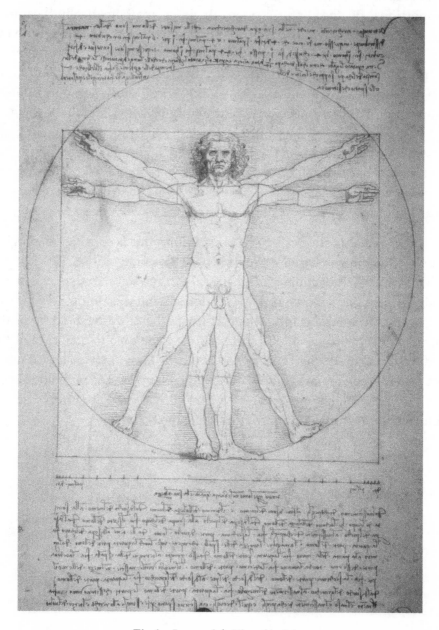

Fig 1. Leonardo's Vitruvian Man

Adaptive Immune system

About 3.5 billion years ago, our home planet is said to have sprung to life. Like all planets, it started as a collection of stardust and the force of gravity, which compacted it to the form we see today, with a hot boiling lava core and a surface of land and oceans that allowed life to flourish. The planet's evolution is well understood, and science has a clear historical development of events that generate our Earth and its moon. Life on Earth, however, is a different story. There are several credible theories that predict that life traveled to our planet from outer space. An asteroid—which contains ice—can easily bring life from distant areas of the universe to our planet. Some postulate that we were seeded by life from Mars, which has now been found to have traces of water. Whether or not you believe that life started on Earth, or that it came from outer space, what is well understood is that life grew from a single-cell organism into a more complex multi-cell organism—this is the theory of evolution. This evolution of our multicellular bodies tells the story of the Adaptive Immune System (AIS).

Multicellular organisms, metazoans, started about 600 million years ago. The planet had an oxygen-rich environment during this time, and life seems to have exploded during this period, so much so that scientists called the period the "evolutionary big bang." Our innate immunity got its origin from these early eukaryotes, cells that contain a nucleus and organelles, and are enclosed by a plasma membrane. Examples are protozoa—single-cell eukaryotic organisms—plants, animals, and fungi. Eukaryotic cells are larger and more complex than prokaryotic cells, which are found in Archaea and Bacteria—the other two forms of life. One early form of eukaryotic life is the amoeba. The amoebas, with their see-through bodies and single-cell organism, are ideal for studying the cell mechanism and processes. When they feed, one can see what looks like an early form macrophage—a type of blood cell of the immune system, cells that engulf and digest pathogens—at work. The AIS in eukaryotes comes from the urge of unicellular microorganisms such as amoeba to discriminate between food, itself, and other amoebas. Without this mechanism, they will eat themselves and will create their own extinction. The mechanism that gives the amoebas the ability to differentiate between food, itself, and other forms of biomass, pathogens, is similar, we can infer, to the most basic function of the immune system. The immune system needs to know when it is under attack; it must destroy only the invader, not itself or its host. Like macrophages, amoebas move around randomly, unless they detect an invader; then, they head in the same direction to eliminate the threat. All animals have a population of phagocytic cells in their immune system which patrol the body, and which have much in common with amoebas.

Innate immunity is the type of immunity with which we are born. Acquired immunity, on the other hand, refers to enhancements to the immune system—by nature and or environmental conditions. We fight specific viruses and develop immunity; this development is adaptive or acquired immunity. The immune system is charged with fighting what the body considers pathogens or foreign bodies that can harm the body. When this system is in a healthy state, the response to attack is fast and efficient. Those people that focus on optimizing their immune system seldom get sick and, if they do, they recover rather quickly. This is equivalent to have a strong army in a city that is being attacked. If the army is efficient and in good health, it will quickly dispose of the enemy. This city will rarely get attacked and, in those instances in which it does, victory is certain most of the time.

The AIS is a network of cells, organs, and feedback loops that are essential to maintain human health. It protects the body from microorganisms like bacteria, viruses, and fungi. When these enter the body, the AIS goes into battle mode and quickly disposes of the invaders, if one has a strong system. While in the heat of battle, the body may feel side effects like fever, sweating, and other signs which warn us that the body is being attacked. Since the body is self-healing and self-regulating, it is imperative that we allow the body enough time to do this healing without medical intervention. As we experience the first sign of fever or high temperature, we immediately reach for the over the counter medication. A fever is a way the body deals with most pathogen attacks since these are not able to survive at high temperatures. When we rush to lower our internal body temperature, we are overriding this mechanism and not allowing the body to get stronger. The next time that same pathogen attacks, the body will not be properly prepared. We have an over-reliance on drugs and medication, which are loaded with side effects. These drugs are efficient at dealing with symptoms — for example, by reducing the temperature or minimizing the pain — but they do not address the real root cause of illness in the first place. It is important that we constantly "train" our AIS and give it the best natural nutrition and exercise to reach its peak performance. Without a strong AIS, the body cannot reach its full health potential. Factors that can decrease the performance of the AIS include chronic stress, inadequate nutrition, exposure to environmental toxins, smoking, and obesity.

❧

White cells, also known as leukocytes, are the primary soldiers the AIS uses to fight harmful pathogens. These cells circulate all over the body via blood vessels and lymphatic vessels, patrolling for foreign invaders. When they encounter a pathogen, they start to multiply and, they start to send signals to other cells of the AIS, alerting them of the attack. The white cells are stored in the lymphoid organs. These include the thymus, spleen, lymph nodes, and bone marrow. In addition to these organs, we also find other issues — like tonsils, skins, and membranes of throat, nose, and genitals — also play a role in the storage and support of the immune system. The key to the immune response is to manage the relationship between antibody and antigen (antigen is an invader microorganism). When the AIS recognizes an antigen, it produces antibodies. Types of antibodies — a type of immunoglobulins — are proteins that attach specific antigens to protect the body. These antibodies are very specialized and each antibody attacks specific antigens, such as bacteria and other microbes. By understanding all these components, systems, and processes, one can keep them in peak performance and one can give the AIS the best fighting chance to win over any illness or foreign microbes' attack. Consequently, optimum health can be attained when one has a strong immune system. The AIS can also breakdown. It may fail to protect the body if it is damaged in some way. Obesity, excessive alcohol, and a toxic lifestyle are just a few of the factors that can contribute to a weak immune system. Autoimmune disorders like rheumatoid arthritis cause the immune system to mistake the body's own tissues as invaders. Some key factors to optimize your immune body system are:

- **Regular exercise:** at least 4 or 5 times a week for at least 45 minutes (always consult your doctor before you start any exercise program).
- **Meditation:** Oxygenation of the body, relaxation of all muscles, lowering of all stress levels are just a few of the benefits of meditation.
- **Proper nutrition:** giving the cells of your body the natural ingredients they need to grow, thrive, and multiply.
- **Laughter:** Laughter is another form of relaxation that is highly effective at reducing your stress level. Remember that stress is one of the main causes of all your ills.
- **Stress management:** being able to reduce or eliminate all sources of stress.

CHAPTER 3: STATE OF BEING

NATURAL BODY STATE—ADAPTIVE FITNESS

Health is a relationship between you and your body.

— Anonymous

I n 1856, a relatively unknown monk was conducting experiments by crossbreeding pea plants of different phenotypes to determine how, if any, changes were being passed on to related pea plants. His experiment would change the course of genetics. Gregor J. Mendel, known as the "father of modern genetics," is mostly known for this famous experiment, breeding peas and using them to gather data about what he would later call dominant and recessive genes.

Mendel was born in Heinzendorf, at the Moravian-Silesian Border — now the Czech Republic. He was one of three siblings and was raised on a small farm. Young Mendel worked as a gardener and studied beekeeping. His family, financially strapped, struggled to pay for his studies. He studied physics and philosophy at the Philosophical Institute of the University of Olomouc. The Department of Philosophy was headed by Johann Nestler who, at the time, was doing research on hereditary traits of plants and animals. This may have influenced young Mendel. Following a recommendation from his teacher, Mendel entered the Augustinian St. Thomas' Abbey and began his training as a priest. Joining a monastery may be odd to us now, but it was not unusual during his time. Monasteries have several functions during this time; in addition to being places of prayer and worship, they had to be self-sufficient. They grew their food, made cheese, wine, and assisted the poor. Monasteries were also often places of intellectual activities. Mendel wanted to be a teacher, but he failed his exam for certification, not once but twice. After taking some additional formal education, he eventually passed the certification and returned to the monastery as a teacher of physics. As a monk in the monastery, Mendel had access to an experimental garden in which he would breed different colors and kinds of peas, and he meticulously recorded all possible combinations. His experiments involved growing thousands of pea plants for a period of eight years. He isolated several parameters, like plant height, pod shape, and color. His results showed that, when a yellow pea and a green were bred together, their offspring plant was always yellow. However, in the next generation of plants, the green peas reappeared at a ratio of 1:3. To explain his result, Mendel coined the term: "recessive" and "dominant" in reference to certain traits. Mendel had no concept of genes as we know them today, but his groundbreaking work set up the road to our current understanding of heredity and genes. He published his work in 1866, showing the effect of "invisible factors" which we now call genes.

Mendel was never recognized during his life for his accomplishment. It took more than three decades, after his death, for his discoveries to be truly recognized as the milestone they were. His pea study established many of the rules of heredity now referred to as the laws of "Mendelian inheritance." Mendel was the first to describe dominant and recessive traits that can be transferred from parent to offspring. He also described the heterozygote and homozygote. Homozygous refers to having identical alleles for a single trait. An allele represents one particular form of a gene. In addition, he pinpointed the difference between genotype and phenotype. Genotype refers to the genetic make-up of a species, while phenotype refers to the visible traits.

⌒⌒⌒

Darwin used the Gemmule to describe a microscopic unit of inheritance. This would later be known as chromosomes; however, chromosomes were first observed during cell division by Wilhelm Hofmeister, as early as 1848. Hofmeister, a Danish botanist, coined the word "gene" to describe a fundamental physical and functional unit of heredity. William Bateson, in 1905, coined the term genetics from the word gene. The actual mechanism of how the gene operated and passed the information cargo was not yet completely understood. By 1941, George Wells Beadle and Edward Lawrie Tatum proposed the "one gene" hypothesis. This hypothesis states that genes act through the production of enzymes, with each gene responsible for producing a single enzyme that in turn affects a single step in a metabolic pathway. The understanding of the genes as a function of change took a giant leap when in 1953, James Watson and Francis Crick were trying to put together a model of DNA and end it up discovering the double helix structure of the DNA molecule. This discovery would get them both the Nobel Prize for Medicine.

The genes, through the process of natural selection and random mutation, are responsible for the myriad of phenotypes that we see around us. Nature records successful traits and passes these on to the next generation. This is a natural process. With our current advances in genetics, we are learning how to manipulate the genes, and we are starting to bioengineer our own genome. The Human Genome Project was completed in 2003. The researchers managed to map all the genes of the human body; the Genome Project estimated that humans have between 20,000 and 25,000 genes. This was a gigantic feat and led the way towards the understanding of our design and the possibility of starting to understand how all our genes really work and what areas they are affecting. The Genome Project is more like a blueprint for building a human. Changes to our genome are also generated by the environmental factors, without changing the actual DNA gene structures. A change in phenotype without a change in genotype is referred to as epigenetics changes – the genes are turned on and off. Epigenetics is the study of heritable changes in gene expression – active versus inactive genes – that do not involve changes to the underlying DNA sequence. Epigenetic changes, by nurture, are naturally occurring and can have a significant effect on the body. The environment, your lifestyle, and your overall health state all can produce epigenetic changes that can manifest as serious illnesses and be passed on to offspring. Cancer was one of the first human diseases to be linked to epigenetics. Studies have shown that prenatal and early postnatal environmental factors can influence adult risk of developing various forms of chronic diseases and behavioral disorders. The tragic event that, in 1944-45, led to the Dutch Hunger Winter famine – in which a large segment of the population had little to nothing to eat – created a unique opportunity to study the relationship between prenatal famine and health in adult life. This period of malnutrition created epigenetic changes in the population that were passed to the children. Studies have shown that the children born during the Dutch Hunger Winter famine have increased rates of coronary heart disease and obesity when compared to those children not exposed to the famine. Adults that were prenatally exposed to famine conditions have also been reported to have a significantly higher incidence of schizophrenia. The environment is a powerful influence on epigenetic changes and disease susceptibility. Pollution, for example, could alter the methyl tags on DNA – turn genes on – and increase one's risk for neurodegenerative diseases.

Nature and nurture—Homo sapiens adaptation duo

Fitness – the state of being physically fit and healthy – birthed out of our natural necessity to survive in a highly competitive and dangerous environment. Eat or be eaten – only the fittest survive. According to the United States Department of Health and Human Services, a person is fit if she has a good level of physical fitness and has a set of attributes that people have or achieve that relates to the ability to perform physical activity. However, this set of attributes only addresses a single area of fitness, the physical aspect. An all-encompassing definition of fitness needs to consider all aspects affecting the entirety of the body — its muscular structures and performance, its ability to function optimally for the selected environment, and the mental and happiness state. This is the holistic approach to fitness. Since the body and the mind are intimately connected, one cannot engage in fitness discourse without considering both components. When we study animals in the wild, we rarely observe animals that are not fit or are "fat" for their living environment. If they are, natural selection will ensure that they are not able to reproduce, and they eventually will fall to predation and or competition. The survival of the fittest ensures that the optimum genes survive and are passed to future generations. Hence, animals living in a natural environment, eating their regular diet, are the closest to their ideal physical fitness level.

Environmental changes and random mutations ensure that the animal is constantly adapting to new conditions and improving to cope with ever-changing living conditions and pressures. Their state of well-being is a natural one in which they have the optimal physical capability to reproduce, survive, and preserve the species and themselves. We are higher evolved animals. Our highly developed cerebral cortex endows us with the capacity to learn and pass this knowledge to our offspring. This single advantage has been enough to propel us to the top of the food chain. However, we are still animals, and our physical fitness, like the animals mentioned above, is at optimum, as well, when we are in concert with nature and when we are living in harmony with our environment. In addition to this concern, we have a consciousness and a mind that demands fitness, as well. The mental aspect of fitness is as important as the physical one, and they work in concert to maintain the whole, fit and content. If either one breaks down, then the whole system breaks down. A natural body is one that follows natural diets, consumes real food, engages in physical activities that mirror living in nature, activities that our ancestors performed, like running, playing, etc. It follows, then, that being in tune with nature is paramount to overall health and happiness. S natural state refers to a state in which we are living as close as to nature as possible. This will entail, by logical deduction, being as far as possible from artificial environments and products. The natural state is what organisms were designed by nature to do. Genetic changes passed down by inheritance, gene mutations, and epigenetic changes caused by the environment; all combine to create the variations we see in the human genus. Consider what we eat: are these foods "artificially" or synthetically created? Consider when one sits in an office environment for eight hours a day: was the body "naturally designed" for this monotonous and repetitive task? Humans' natural existence and relationship with the natural world are key parameters on the road to fitness. The terms "artificial" will be used in this book to denote artifacts that are created by man—Genetically Modified Organism (GMO), cosmetics, packaged goods, processed foods, etc. Technically, everything is natural as all chemical elements exist in nature, and everything is made of elements, but for the purpose of this discussion, we will consider artificial those alterations made by man and mostly driven by profit motives. Natural will be used to refer to products made by nature and the natural selection processes. Nature and the process of natural selection is a terribly slow process as it takes thousands of years, and sometimes millions of years, to produce a winning trait. Natural evolution is a slow, methodical, and highly efficient process as it considers all the parameters that affect the particular element being optimized. On insects and other animals with a short lifespan, this process is relatively shorter. Fruit flies, for example, have multiple generations in a matter of weeks, but even in this case, nature does not produce phenotype change at high speed. Nature has taken millions of years to optimally design our exquisite, complex human body. The human design information is passed along by the genes—the unit of currency for biological changes—and these take multiple generations to produce changes that will last and become winning traits.

Evolution is the ultimate optimizer because it considers every single factor, parameters that influence the species being evolved. In the development of the human body, nature considers every possible interaction with millions of chemicals, and with trillions of microorganisms, and their combination. This level of complexity and these combinations of factors are not possible to model with our current state of technology, as the combinations will require computational power not available at this time. The scientific approach to this problem is to approximate an answer by limiting the number of parameters and using "approximations." The iterative nature of this process—evolving our human body—is then slow, methodical, and highly optimized. Nature and nurture, working the genes, epigenetics, and the forces of the environment, all have combined to create that which is you. An optimized state is obtained due to trial and error, and by only keeping the "best optimum solution" for future generations. The process of mutation and or adaptation, natural selection, and the changes due to the current environment all meet to create the optimal state. It is this process that creates an optimum state of fitness. Note, however, that not all genotypes take that long to develop, but time is always a key factor.

Nature likes to take its time to ensure the benefits are worth that effort. If we consider the hardware and software analogy, the body is the hardware part of this duality, and the environment is the software. It follows, then, that to be fit, to operate at the highest possible level, one will need to have the best hardware available. This hardware is not purchased at the store but, instead, is inherited from our parents, and mother nature plays its part to adapt the genes. We can mold, reshape, and constantly upgrade the software through our interaction with the environment—nurturing. If we exercise, have proper nutrition, and reduce the level of our stress, we are rewarded with the best available software for our body. Additionally, as we learned above, the hardware can be modified, as well, as the epigenetics changes—turning genes on and off—modify the functions of our genes. It is this combination of nature and nurture that we can manipulate to ensure that our bodies are optimized to the environment. In upcoming chapters, we will expand how we can induce these epigenetic changes to remake our bodies into the best version of what we can be. Specifically, the design of our way of eating, proper exercise, rest, and toxic elimination will be a few of the items that we will explore to start changing our body and epigenetic design. The body is in its best fitness when it is in tune with nature. One must realize that one is part of a grand plan, that one is intimately connected to all, and nature is the canvas where we create life. To be in tune with nature means to live in a natural way, as much as possible, avoiding artificial foods, toxic exposures, and harmful environments. Naturally fit is eating natural, plant-based wholesome food, avoiding exposure to toxins and harsh chemicals, and reducing all forms of stress.

The optimum physique—natural, muscular, and proportional

A body in a natural environment is endowed with the optimal muscular structure to survive and multiply. This is natural selection at work. If an animal's physical structure does not allow him to fight for food, avoid predation, and or reproduce, it will go extinct. Therefore, animals in the wild have the optimum structure. Humans are animals as well; the main difference is that our highly evolved brains have allowed us to circumvent these natural challenges with our wit and intelligence. Our brain concocted ways to store food, create surplus, and design processes and procedures aimed at improving the survival and reproduction of the species. It also invented the use of tools, which eventually replaced the need for physical laboring as the main source of survival. The artificial environment of modern living took over more and more of the natural ways of early man and, by eliminating all the needs for the physical requirement to survive, it made the body weaker in return. We are headed in the USA to obesity levels of one in two in just a year or so. By abandoning the ways of our earlier ancestors and by not replacing the physical demands used in time past, lives have become sedentary. A body in a natural state is a body in a state of health.

The power output of the body reflects your muscular structure. Muscular composition dictates how much work one can put out. Think of a car with an exceptionally large engine – high horsepower. It would be able to do a lot more work than an equivalent size car with a smaller engine. The muscular composition can be evaluated based on the body fat percentage, an efficiency metric, its muscle size, and definition – a power metric. All features of living organisms are evolved by "optimizing" all parameters relevant to the survival and reproduction of the organism. These all come pre-programmed with one prime objective in mind: to reproduce and preserve itself. Consider homo sapiens' muscle size: if the muscles were bigger, this would give her a competitive advantage and allow her to go over bigger size prey, but it comes at a cost. The larger muscles require higher amounts of energy and slow her down when chasing faster pray. The optimum size for the muscle is the one that gives her the maximum advantage in consideration of the energy expenditure for the given environmental conditions. This is a very fluid evolution and it is constantly changing to produce the optimum state. So, we can conclude that having the largest muscle in the group is not the optimum state because it depends on the environmental conditions. A smaller size of muscle will allow her to chase a higher pool of prey. One logical deduction from the above argument is that nature dictates the optimum condition better than any other artificial mechanism. Nature takes an iterative, slow, and long-term process to come up with the optimum size. Now, consider a modern weightlifter who has worked to get her body to reach the level of growth way above that of the average individual. This individual has reached muscular structures that severely limit her range of motion and also limit her ability to produce explosive power. By consuming an unnaturally high number of calories, and sometimes supplements, and growth-inducing hormones, she has amassed a very heavy, oversized muscular structure.

We are familiar with this type of muscular body type since we awe at the muscle size of these individuals and reward the top of these individuals with trophies and monetary awards. This individual is not optimized for their environment. Their mobility is severely limited, and they can certainly not chase any type of prey or run from a dangerous situation for any significant amount of time. Because of the heavy weight of their bodies, they have traded athletic performance for muscular size. Although we no longer need to chase our food on the savanna — thanks to the advent of supermarkets — we still are required to maintain a healthy level of flexibility and speed to escape from danger and sometimes to avoid it. Many of these overweight individuals end up with a myriad of medical conditions like enlarged hearts, cancers, kidney failure, and so on, just to name a few. Notice that I am looking at the end-range individual on this sports spectrum only. The average weightlifter that can perform a high level of aerobic exercise and is highly mobile is not included in this category. A "natural" optimization of weight takes into consideration all aspects of interacting with the environment: such as the ability to run, endurance, speed, cardio health, and interaction with others of the same species. An overall muscular physique is a competitive advantage and allows us to mate more easily – reproduction, to take care of ourselves (safety) and our families, and to live healthier and pain-free due to the muscular support structure.

There are 650 muscles in the human body. We must work on each one of them constantly to keep our bodies in the best possible shape. A muscular, symmetrical body is one that we can obtain if we work at it and make a goal to acquire it. Regardless of our age, this is an attainable goal. We know of centenarians who are very physically active, whose bodies still show a very defined muscular structure, capable of producing a copious amount of work. The development of the muscular body begets the strong immune system and consequently, the ability to resist diseases. Our immune system is directly related to our physical state. If we have a low-fat body with high levels of muscular structures, then it follows that we will have a strong immune system as well. Since this system is responsible for fighting pathogens and keeping us in a healthy state, then a muscular body is a healthy body. We must strive to achieve the highest possible level of muscular definition and muscle size while at the same time also increasing our ability to do work – cardiovascular performance.

By training for strength, flexibility, and stamina, we can achieve all of these. Nature and nurture give us all the performance parameters we need to succeed. Our target should include as well increase our output performance. The performance referred to here is more associated with the power or capacity to perform a given task in each time interval. Consider, for example, the ability to run a mile under four minutes. That is a very specific performance. We can train to increase this performance – by reducing the time in which we complete the mile. As it relates to holistic fitness, performance includes flexibility, strength, and stamina. In a natural environment, a high-performance animal is one who risks his life in order to feed himself and his family and to avoid predation and any other forms of danger. Individuals are at optimum performance when they can reach the maximum level for their given environment and physiological condition. It is the combination of three metrics, flexibility, strength, and stamina, that determines the overall level of performance. If one has incredible flexibility but is unable to sustain a high level of physical activity for a long time, then one will not be considered a fit individual. The value range for these parameters was reviewed in Part Two. Stamina measures cardiovascular health combined with muscular strength. Cardiovascular endurance indicates how well the body can provide fuel during physical activities, using the circulatory and respiratory system. Maintaining physical fitness will help prevent most diseases.

A fit body is a muscular and proportional body. Muscle size is not as important as proportionally built muscles, which optimizes the amount of work that a person can do. A professional weightlifter, for example, has a body that is not efficiently designed to perform a maximum amount of work. Nature optimizes the body so that it is not too small or too large; it is just perfect for the given environment. A cross-fit professional athlete, for example, has a body that is optimally designed to do the maximum amount of work. He can perform cardio exercises as well as strength exercises in the optimal range for humans.

Natural body state—illness-free state

Dr. John Bergman often argues that diseases do not really exist. He advocates promoting health instead of fighting diseases. He argues that, if one changes one's belief system, if one does not listen to all the non-scientific, nonsensical advice of some well-intentioned doctors who, unfortunately, have been indoctrinated in their profession with outdated medical practices, and if one takes care of one's body, then diseases will start to disappear as the body can heal itself. One example of ill-advised mentality is the obsession with over cleaning and sterilizing everything we come in contact with. The medical industry has convinced the general public that washing your hands as frequently as possible, sterilizing all the surfaces in your house, and killing bacteria everywhere one finds it, is absolutely critical to good health. They will have you believe that playing on the dirt is not good or that being exposed to pathogens is extremely dangerous. Over-prescription of antibiotics is a result of this mindset. The problem with this advice is that we are made of mostly bacteria! When we kill these bacteria, we are making ourselves sick.

Our guts – our microbiota – for example, contain tens of trillions of microorganisms, including at least 1000 different species of known bacteria with more than 3 million genes, 150 times more than human genes. It is believed that about two-thirds of these microorganisms are very specific to the individual, a form of ID card. The gut sometimes is referred to as a second brain. It contains some 100 million neurons, more than in either the spinal cord or the peripheral nervous system. Most of one serotonin – a neurotransmitter involved in the role of emotions and happiness – is produced in the gut, about 90%. One way to promote health is to feed our microbiome – the gut community of microorganisms that keeps us healthy. Our microbiome is responsible for the bulk of our immune system, our pathogen defense system. The best way to stay healthy is by making our immune system as strong as possible. This is accomplished by feeding the microbiome the correct set of nutrients, enough to keep the community of microorganisms on the gut healthy and growing. When the person is in optimal shape, they do not get sick or, if they do, the illness only lasts a few days. The reason is that a natural body is primed to fight infections. It has all the muscle, immune system, and stress-free state needed to successfully fight pathogens. Illness should be thought of as a transitional stage that reminds the individual of what the healthy states feel like. This line of reasoning views the positive side of illness – it is just a path on the way to wellness, and it also helps one appreciate a totally healthy state.

There are some key major trends that are producing chronic diseases in modern society. Antibiotic over-prescription is making the body weak by also killing the good bacteria as well as promoting the development of "super-bugs" or microorganisms that are immune to antibiotics. Babies delivered by Caesarean section are also deprived of the immune system strength they would get have had they been born vaginally. The birth channel contains the mother's biota that the baby can inherit if it is born vaginally. Other trends producing illness is city-living: crowded conditions and closeness, with a lack of natural environmental exposure. With no room to experience the outdoors, city-dwelling individuals are victims of their artificial environment. One final trend to notice is the overuse of prescription drugs. Modern living is becoming synonymous with using drugs to cure any and all ills. The body is rarely given an opportunity to practice self-healing. A state of being illness-free is the natural state, but it can only be obtained by eliminating all these trends.

PART TWO: THE SECOND NOBLE TRUTH

Stress-free is Thy Answer

We build too many walls and not enough bridges.

—Sir Isaac Newton

N o discourse on the topic of "stress" or forces would be complete without the mention of Sir Isaac Newton—the father of modern science. He was a physicist and mathematician in England in the sixteen century. His works are the foundations of physics, engineering, calculus, and he is also credited with jump-starting the scientific revolution. Newton's equations of motion allow us to put a man on the moon, to design modern computers, to build bridges, and to design almost any conceivable modern consumer product. Classical mechanics is called Newtonian physics to honor his name.

Newton was born on Christmas Day—December 25, 1642— an hour or two after midnight, at the Woolsthorpe Manor, in Woolsthorpe-by-Colsterworth, in the county of Lincolnshire, England. His father—Isaac

Newton, whom he was named after—had died three months earlier. Newton was born prematurely, to a poor family. His mother, Hannah Ayscough, would later say of the birth that "Newton could have fit inside a quart mug." She remarried by the time Newton reached three-years of age and moved to live with her new husband, the Reverend Barnabas Smith, leaving young Newton in the care of his maternal grandmother, Margery Ayscough. He disliked his stepfather and would later confess in a list of sins to "threatening my father and mother Smith to burn them and the house over them." Newton, while a teenager, went to school at The King's School, Grantham, which taught Latin, Greek, and likely impart in him the foundation for his mathematics. In 1659, his mother removed him from school, after her second husband passed, and try to make a farmer out of him—an occupation he hated. The schoolmaster, Henry Stokes, convinced his mother to bring him back to school. It is said that, motivated by revenge against schoolyard bullies, he became the top-ranked student and distinguished himself mostly by building sundials and windmills.

In 1661, he was admitted to Trinity College, Cambridge, based on a recommendation of his uncle Rev. William Ayscough, who was an Alumni of the school. He was able to secure scholarships until he was awarded his degree. The teachings of the time were based on the works of Aristotle, Descartes, Galileo, and Kepler. By 1665, he discovered the generalized binomial theorem and began to develop the mathematical theories that would later become calculus. Soon after he got his BA degree, the university temporarily closed as a precaution against the Great Plaque. His home studies during these times resulted in the development of his theories on calculus, optics, and the law of gravitation. Soon after, he returned to Trinity College as an elected fellow. Fellows were required to become ordained priests, but this was not enforced during the years of restoration. When this issue came back again a few years later, Newton was able to avoid it by getting special permission from King Charles II. His studies at Trinity were highly impressive and by 1669 Newton was elected a Fellow of the Royal Society and became a Lucasian professor—this chair is considered the most renowned academic chair in the world. In 1703, he was elected as president of the Royal Society. He was knighted by Queen Anne in 1705. Newton died in 1727, at the age of 84. His work totally consumed him and, sadly, he never married.

⁌

It is said that on a cool crisp morning, a curious youngster – while walking on an apple orchard – meticulously observed an apple fall to the ground. This event has been witnessed thousands of times before by many, but this time it was different; now it was being observed instead of just being looked at. "Why is the apple falling down? It is as if it were being pulled down by an invisible string." "What is it making it go down?" "Do all apples fall at the same speed – does size matter?" To the layman, this mere act is insignificant. There is nothing special about things falling. Everything falls. "What's special about this apple?" The youngster was none other than the giant of science, Sir Isaac Newton. The simple act of an apple falling to the ground would have been of no significance to anyone, as this act has been seen thousands of times before, but this time the act was being observed by Newton. With unrelenting devotion and scientific questioning, he went on to explain why apples and any other objects fall to the ground. He would not only postulate the law of gravity but would describe the laws of motion in physics in such an outstanding clarity that more than four hundred years later, we are still using his laws to send humans into space and do all engineering solutions.

Isaac Newton's three laws of motion, *"Philosophiae Naturalis Principia Mathematica,"* were first published in 1687. Recall that we defined stress as a normalized force (or a force per unit area). Newton's law will tell us the nature of forces – including gravity – and their action on masses. Given this force, we can determine the physical stress related to the force (i.e., by simply applying this force on the area in which it is acting). A broken bone, a torn skin, a pinched nerve, are examples of physical stress when a force, physical in nature, acts on them to cause a fracture or strain. Newtonian physics allows us to calculate the stress (and force) associated with the failure. This is the physics we see every day, and it will assist us in understanding where the physical stress on the body comes from. Newton laws of motion are today the fundamental principles of engineering, and they are used to design products, calculate stresses, determine failure points, and for countless other mathematical and scientific applications. Physical stresses are based on these fundamental principles. Newton's law of motion can be stated as:

- *Every object in a state of uniform motion will remain in that state of motion unless an external force acts on it.*
- *Force equals mass times acceleration.*
- *For every action, there is an equal and opposite reaction.*

Motion is the result of potential differences. Two electric poles with different charges, for example, will generate a current on an electric circuit. A river will flow from its highest point to its lowest. The wind will travel from a point of low pressure to a point of high pressure. When a system is in total equilibrium, there is nothing happening on it; it is a motionless state of death. Without difference, there cannot be motion — motion generates force — then there cannot be force either. Stress is a force normalized over area — hence, whenever there is a force present, there is stress. Forces in life abound. Physical, chemical, and mental forces all produce the stresses we experience daily. Maladies are just breakdowns — higher than normal stresses of the body. All maladies are the results of some form of stress or a combination of stresses.

CHAPTER 4: AS A MATTER OF HARMONY

STRESS—NATURE AND ORIGIN

Every human being is the author of his own health or disease

— Buddha

A discourse on stress will be incomplete if its colloquial meanings on mundane conversations are excluded. Stress in a regular conversation is, in many instances, ambiguous and people, in general, do not have a common understanding of it—consequently, its uses get diluted; the message is confusing and ineffective. In street conversation, one hears: "I have a lot of stress," "I am so stressed," "you stress me so much!" and "I cannot take the stress." These meanings equate stress to an object that gets passed from one person to another; however, stress is not a thing, it is a state. Engineering has a very precise definition of stress, which is what is meant when we use stress in a scientific matter. To ensure accuracy of communication, we will refer to stress in this manner, as a state of stress or when a system is acted upon by a "force". Stress defined as force per unit area will also be used for all forms of stress, whether it is mental, chemical, or physical. The force component of stress will change depending on the force being used. A system under stress has a point at which it fails or breaks; this is sometimes referred to as a "critical" stress or breaking point. There are three fundamental types of stresses that we will explore: physical stress, chemical stress, and mental stress. Further chapters will explore each detail. When the stress level of humans reaches a breaking point, we experience a breakdown, or most commonly called illness or maladies. With this consideration in mind, we can postulate that all maladies are caused by stress, even genetic diseases—in this case, the stress happened in prior generations. The stress associated with the force responsible for its present dictates the type of diseases in questions. Diabetes type 2, for example, caused by insulin resistance on the cell bodies, can be traced back to stress on the cell receptors. If we can think of a hormone acting on a receptor as a key opening a lock, then, one can also think of a force (or stress) as the key and the maladies as the lock. We will use pressure and stress interchangeably. In the English system, we measure pressure as pounds per square inch (or PSI).

> **Stress** /stress/ *noun* 1. Pressure or tension exerted on a material object. 2. A state of mental or emotional strain or tension resulting from adverse or very demanding circumstances.

For example, typical tire pressure is about 35 psi. To understand the effect of stress, then it follows that we must first find the source of the force responsible for the stress. Additionally, we need to consider where the force action resides. These two factors combined will give a general picture of the stress involved.

A mischievous young boy, Cheme, is climbing an ancient apple tree. As he gets higher up the tree and gazes at the ground, now so far below, his enthusiasm gets the best of him. A snap of a fragile branch sends him tumbling down the tree—passing already conquered tree limbs—and finally smashing loudly and spectacularly on the hard ground below. The fall breaks not only the little boy's femur bone but his pride as well. These types of fractures are mechanical failure in nature, as the force involved is a mechanical force—the impact of the fall due to gravity. Stress has two basic components: force and area. The force component of stress is relatively easy to locate. In the case of Cheme's fracture, the force can be calculated using simple Newtonian physics and the momentum created by the fall. This is mechanical stress on his bone, that was high enough to go surpass its critical stress. The force itself has a direction and can cause the object in question to bend, twist, compress, or expand. There are infinite numbers of ways that a force can be applied to an object. In scientific discourse, we clearly state the nature of the force and the stress state of the object being investigated. Compression stress tells us that the force exerted on the system is of compressive nature. Imagine a bridge during heavy rush hour traffic. All the cars riding over the bridge will exert a force pushing the bridge down; this will result in a bridge under compressive stress. The same bridge can be under tension force as its own weight is trying to stretch the bridge down to the ground. This language for stress is a scientific and very precise way to refer to stress. One can extend this use of stress definition to the human body, its psychology, and its medical applications. Let us consider a spine under stress. It would be ambiguous if we just say that the spine is under stress. To make a valuable inference and hopefully to eliminate all stresses, we need to understand what the source of stress is. Is the force a compressive load? Or is the spine arch too much? Is it under chemical load? It is not enough to say it is under stress as this does not specify the origin of the stress load. If the spine is "curved," then we can say the force is tension in some areas—the outside part of the spine—and compression on the inside part. As knowledgeable and educated consumers, we must seek the true root cause of any stress. Next time one visits the doctor and she says one is under high stress, challenge her to explain what the source of the stress is, what is the force that is causing this stress? If she cannot answer, then it is time to get a second opinion. Only by knowing the root causes of stress can one hope to eradicate it.

Life is like riding a bicycle. To keep your balance you must keep moving.

— Albert Einstein

Stress, focused force

Whenever you have a force acting on a body, you will have stress. Since forces come from an infinite number of sources, it follows that stress also comes from infinite sources. All forces in nature can be grouped into four fundamental forces: the weak force, strong force, electromagnetism, and gravity. All matter is made from fundamental particles, and particles are governed by these fundamental forces. It follows then that all matter is only acted upon by just these four forces. To simplify the discourse, we will use the general terms of everyday language for these forces — like wind force, water pressure, weight, and so on. However, one must keep in mind that all forces can be boiled down to just those four above. It is a significant and a great triumph of science that we can narrow down the whole universe interactions to just four basic forces. These four forces are responsible for keeping every atom together, for keeping us on the ground, for galaxy formation, for every cell and biological unit action, and for every single action and reaction in the universe.

Fundamental forces are expanded to groups that we can relate to in daily life. We talk about thermal force or chemical force without detailing their fundamental component. This is prudent as it will simplify the discussion at hand. It is important, however, to realize that all forces are a subset of the fundamental forces. Consider the nature of the stress of a living biological organism. It is under several pressures coming from interacting with its environment. The outer layer of one's skin — epidermis — experiences surface stress. It is under stress from all forces that it meets, like wind, water, other organisms, regular matter, and many others. Any contact with the environment results in some stress. The

61

nature of the interaction will dictate the type of force involved: electromagnetic, weak, and strong, and so on. The epidermis could be pushed, pulled, squeezed, and or twisted, depending on the origin of the interaction, and then a stress level would follow. The stress level will also depend on the strength of the force being applied. Stress is always present when one thinks of it in this fashion, as there is always a type of force acting on the system. If you have "no force" acting on the system, then it will expand forever without bound, as there is no force to stop it from expanding. Stress is then a relative quantity. Since stress is always present in one form or another, then the stress level, and how close it is to the breaking point, becomes key. If the stress is too high—higher than the critical stress for the object in question—then the object will fail or break. When we consider a living organism, stress is hyper important to the healthy development of the organism. It is the stress that makes the organism get stronger, grow, and develop its immune system. As one moves around in one's busy life, one is exposed daily to all kinds of stress: physical, mental, and chemical. These stresses and our response to them define whether the individual will become a happy, productive member of society or a slave to these sources of stress. The sources of stress are too many to list, as every interaction result in a force being created which, in turn, means some level of stress. The important ones are those that get excessively high. Physical stress resulting from lack of muscle, misalignment of body posture, weak bone structures, are all examples of typical forces in the physical realm. Keep in mind that stress, in itself, is not bad; on the contrary, it is a necessity of life. However, it must be managed and kept at appropriate levels to be of benefit to the individual.

Maladies—Stress-induced

Any stress that acts on the body tilts it "out of balance." When the body balance—homeostasis— is tilted too far from balance, then disease happens. This view of diseases assumes the body works best under a specific range of conditions, so the breakdown is assumed when the individual is out of its safe range. One tool that is frequently used in quality control to determine the root cause of failure is the "five whys." To use it one would ask why at least five times until one gets to the real root cause of the failure. Let us apply this tool to one of modern society's major epidemic: obesity.

Question 1: *"Why are people obese?"*

Answer: *"Because they consume too many calories and the wrong type of calories."*

Question 2: *"Why do they consume too many calories and the wrong type of calories?"*

Answer: *"Because they are hungry, but they do not understand how nutrition works."*

Question 3: *"Why are they hungry and do not understand nutrition?"*

Answer: *"Their metabolic rate is not optimized and the calories they are consuming are not making them feel full (satiated)."*

Question 4: *"Why is their metabolic rate not optimized and the calories they are consuming are not making them feel full (satiated)?"*

Answer: *"They are not exercising optimally and not getting proper nutrition."*

Question 5: *"Why not?"*

Answer: *"They need to eat properly."*

Notice that with this line of questioning, the answers keep getting progressively better, and one is getting closer to the real root cause of the problem. Today's standard medical approach will stop at the first or second "why." To this question, the standard off-the-shelf medical answer will recommend the standard rehearsed solutions, like surgery to remove fat, or pills to suppress appetite, diets low in fats, and or a combination of all above. This is treating the symptoms, not the real cause of the problem. To effectively resolve the disease, you must ask as many whys as possible until you arrive at the true cause, or the most plausible answer, if the final answer is not known. One should demand a root cause solution to any maladies and not mindlessly accept the standard medical response of just treating the symptoms. A learned individual must understand the causes of the most common conditions that they may face. Far too many people trust their doctor unconditionally. They do not bother to question their authority and wrongly assume that the doctors have all the answers. We are in an era of easy access to information. With a few keystrokes, one can research any condition one desires and get as much information as the doctor has. Most doctors are not trained in nutrition—most medical schools only require 20 hours of nutrition training. Considering how much of a factor nutrition is in good health— that is a good reason not to blindly trust any doctor. One must perform detailed research, question authority, and be the ultimate judge of what's best for one's health. One can also increase one's chance of finding the correct root cause by using DO doctors instead of traditional MD doctors.

Every disease can be traced back to a breakdown of some system, and this, in turn, is due to a force or stress on the system. Therefore, every breakdown or illness is caused by stress. The breakdown can also be a fall off your regular balance, far enough from your normal that it is causing symptoms. We will dig deeper into all types of breakdowns and how these are related to a specific illness. Once you have determined what the root cause or force is that is causing your illness, then you have a chance to address the illness and be completely healed.

To vanish stress, find its source

With the root cause analysis, we can determine the true cause of illness. It is only through this scientific, inquisitive method that we can cure and address the issue of being off-balance, as we look to eliminate the real cause of the disease. Notice, however, that this is not possible all the time. There are some ills for which we do not know the root cause, but we know that stress is involved in the development of the maladies. Stress management will then boil down to just eliminating and or reducing the disease-causing stress from our environment. In situations where we do not know the exact stress causing the illness, a prudent solution would be to reduce and eliminate all the current high-level stresses. This will bring you to your optimum state of happiness and most likely get rid of or reduce the illness.

Allergies, especially around spring when pollen was abundant, affected me badly as I entered my forties. I remember I was unable to be outside for even short periods of time. I would get all the typical symptoms of an allergic reaction: runny nose, red and itchy eyes, sneezing, throbbing headache, and I would feel miserable around this time of the year. My solution at the time was to use an OTC (over the counter) remedy. Zyrtec, an antihistamine, was my medicine of choice and, I would take it religiously during my allergic attacks; within a few days, the symptoms would ease up and eventually disappear. The medication came at a cost since these types of medications have potentially dangerous side effects and can cause memory loss, cognitive impairment, sleep disorders, high blood pressure, diabetes, mood issues, and osteoporosis. Considering all those potentially dangerous side effects, in retrospect, taking this medication was not the right course of action, especially when the solution was so simple. I decided to eliminate this disease and eliminate the need to take any medication, which was full of side effects, many of which were worse than the allergy itself. I started exercising regularly and started training to run my first marathon—a 26.2 mile run. With the exercise regimen came a complete lifestyle change, which includes honey, organic and wholesome foods, a plant-based diet, and avoidance of any processed food. I lost fifty-two pounds during my training and transformed my body in the process. The changes in my immune system were very apparent. The allergies disappeared completely. I never had to touch the allergy medication ever again, and several other benefits came along with the new lifestyle changes like improved memory, improved quality of sleep, more vitality, and overall higher energy. This change in my life convinced me that we could eliminate any disease with the proper lifestyle changes and a positive attitude and outlook on life.

There is more to life than increasing its speed

— Mahatma Gandhi

Profit—driver of stress, engine of growth

Profit is the primary directive of every single company in all our modern societies. The job of every CEO is to "increase shareholder value" or, in other words, to generate profit for the shareholders. A company is a person for legal and tax purposes. A company that does not produce a profit is not going to survive in the long term. Profit is not a bad thing as it is the driver of companies, and it is the force that keeps companies, industries, and people alive and thriving. Companies provide jobs, insurance, financial security, and valuable products and services. The issue becomes when profit is the main driver, and any other social or spiritual concerns are secondary to profit-making. The behavior and actions of the company are consequently driven by optimizing profits because this is the metric of performance that is used to gauge a company. Companies then take this to heart: profitability comes at any cost, and it becomes their prime objective.

This profit-driven mentally is what has produced industries that cloud their benefit to mankind: the tobacco industry, the asbestos industry, Glyphosate (round-up), pesticide and insecticide industries, chemical and pharmaceutical industries, all the industry of pollution, and countless others are examples of where profits come before the health implications of their products. As such, profit then becomes the ultimate social force of modern society. With this insatiable desire to increase profit at all costs, companies are always selling stuff without regard to the actual value their products are producing. A typical teenager is bombarded with thousands of advertisements. It is said that the average American sees or hears over 4,000 ads per day. Advertisers are constantly selling, whether one needs the product or not. It is for this reason that we must keep a healthy dose of skepticism and question every message that is put in front of us. We need to educate ourselves enough to the level where we can judge all these ads and extract the true message: one needs to see beyond the selling pitch. The medical industry is no different than any other industry in the sense that is looking to increase its profit and is selling us on things that we do not need. One needs to study one's body, understand the true nature of diseases, and question any medication and or treatment that doctors recommend. If you have a life-threatening disease, usually you seek a second opinion. You should do the same for any kind of chronic disease or major disease. But for this, we must continue to learn, read constantly, and become better at reading through the lines. Profit as a force, a social driver, is a good way to explain why companies do what they do.

Consider the fast-food industry: clearly, many studies have shown that highly processed foods are nutrient-deficient foods that are, in general, not good for humanity and are a major cause of most chronic diseases. However, unquestionably, these highly processed foods are very "profitable." The fast-food industry is a multi-billion-dollar industry and highly profitable, as the cost of manufacturing these so-called "foods" is incredibly low. In a 2020 Fast Food Analysis Report by the International Franchise Association (IFA), it was reported that globally fast foods generate revenue of over $570 billion per year. In the United States, revenue was $200 billion in 2015, a gigantic increase from the $6 billion in 1970. This trend is clearly increasing, in spite of the obvious adverse health benefits and the increasing prevalence of obesity. The profit-driven force helps explain the motive of these corporations. An educated consumer can see beyond their message and make the correct decision when it comes to selecting what to eat.

The profit-driven force also causes a lot of pressure on those people that are accountable to it. This generates stress throughout the whole value chain. Company workers are stressed, as they need to produce more and more profits; company executives are stressed, as they need to lead the growth; and the trends of profit-driven stress are propagated throughout the entire value chain of product and service. Many employees had felt so much pressure that they had resorted to paying the ultimate price, their lives, when their companies were faced with no profitability, were underperforming and or in bankruptcies. We can use this view of profit to understand many of the trends of modern companies. It explains why some companies continue to push into consumer products that are clearly harmful to the public. Take the sugar industry: the evidence is overwhelming on the adverse effect of refined sugar on the body and, under the banner of providing the customer choices, the sugar industry unapologetically continues to push their product to consumers. Ads from Coke ("open happiness"), Marlboro cigarettes ("Come to where the flavor is"), and a myriad of other deceptive ads are aimed at all audiences to drive sales and to continue to push toxic products to an uninformed public.

Life simplified—stressors vanished

Simplicity is a guiding principle of a happy life. The solution to becoming as healthy as possible is to merely eliminate or reduce all your high-level stressors. There is always going to be a level of stress in one's life; these are needed. The ones to eliminate are the stressors that produce undue, unnecessary, and overly-high stresses. One needs to find the true cause of these and eliminate them at their roots. Simplicity removes things, events, situations, and others, that could potentially be stressors. Consider a very wealthy individual with mansions on several continents. The additional level of responsibility and the need to be aware of what is happening at his properties is enough to raise his personal level of stress.

Simplicity, taken at its core, is an outstanding tool to reduce stressors, eliminate unnecessary burdens, and bring about a simpler, more fulfilling life, where one is focused on what the real priorities. Simplification is sometimes referred to as a "minimalism movement." Although there is no need to take this tool to its extreme, the benefits will become apparent even when used at an average level. Minimizing stress and eradicating stressors are the secret to well-being. When the body is under stress, the body cannot heal. Only when one is in a restful state of mind can one heal.

CHAPTER 5: A PILE OF BROKEN BONES

PHYSICAL STRESS—A STORY OF RESISTANCE

To every action, there is always opposed an equal reaction

— Isaac Newton

M ost of the physical stresses we experience during our daily routines involve some combination of chemical, mental, or physical force. If one looks at a curved spine which is causing undue stress on certain areas due to its curvature and, in addition, it is "pinching" some nerve or squeezing blood carrier vessels, the physical stress in this scenario would be coming from the static and dynamic components of the condition

.

The unnatural curvature produces internal forces that are manifested as stress. Dynamic components arise when motion is added to the area, and the velocities produce forces on the spinal structural members. For every action, there is an equal and opposite reaction. The spine, in this case, is being acted on by a force and, therefore, it is being stressed.

One can also use physical stress in a positive manner to increase the muscles of the body. When a weightlifter is inducing stress on their muscles, due to the weighted exercise they are performing; they are purposely creating stress on the muscles and, since the body is intelligent and self-regulating, it responds by adapting to the added weight by increasing the muscle size. This is the process of gaining muscle by doing weightlifting – positive use of stress to improve body strength and flexibility. In any structure, a simple way to reduce stress is by increasing the strength of the material being used. Then, it follows that if one needs to reduce physical stress, one way one to accomplish it would be by increasing the load-carrying capability of the structural members. The muscular bodies experience lower stress (in general) than a weaker body for the same load. Become stronger and one's physical stress will be reduced.

Physical stress—physicality strained

Physical stress on the body originates from physical forces acting on it. The nature of this load force will determine the reaction of the body. It the load exceeds the body's carrying capability, we then experience fractures, tears, cuts, and structural failure of the member under stress. If the load does not surpass the carrying capacity of the member, then the body only experiences a stretch or compression, depending on the load type. It is critical to understand the source and type of load to be able to assess the type of stress being generated on the body. Most of the pain and discomfort associated with the body are caused by misalignment, improper load carrying, and weak structure bones and muscles.

Consider the stress on the spinal cord, as we evolved from quadruped to bipedal species. The most important aspect of the prehistoric human evolution was the development of bipedalism, which began in primates about four million years ago. This development led to the countless alterations to the human skeleton, including changes to the arrangement and size of the bones of the foot, hip, shape, knee size, leg length, and the shape and orientation of the vertebral column. These evolutionary changes, which happened over millions of years, led to our current body mechanics of the bones and overall body structure. The spine of bipedal Homo sapiens takes a lot of physical stress as it has to withstand higher stresses and endure dynamic force to keep the body in balance. Our muscular structure, as well as the role of the pelvis gurgle, had to change to support the new erect position of the modern human species. A few hypotheses have supported the idea that bipedalism increased the energetic efficiency of travel, and this was a critical factor of bipedal locomotion. Because of this new erect position, human feet evolved enlarged heels to bear the weight of the body. The foot further evolved a foot arch and the smaller size of the toes as compared to ancestors. The human foot transmits weight from the heel, along the outside of the foot and across the ball of the foot and finally to the big toe. This weight transfer yields energy conservation during locomotion. Notice the myriad of new sources of forces due to misalignment, improper posture, foot dynamics, and other locomotion components that can generate physical stress.

The knee, another key source of stress for modern humans, evolved from bipedalism, is enlarged, to better support the increased amount of body weight. Humans walk with their knees straight and thighs bent inward, so that the knees are almost directly under the body, rather than out to the side, as is the case of our ancestral hominids. The spinal cord in humans has a forward bend in the lumbar region and a backward bend in the thoracic region. Without the lumbar curve, the spine would lean forward, a position that needs more effort. With our forward bend, humans use less muscular effort to stand and walk upright. Spinal alignment and spinal stress are also quite common forms of physical stress. Considering all the adaptation that humans evolved into after trying bipedalism, some of the features of the human skeleton remain poorly adapted to bipedalism, leading to negative implications prevalent in humans today. The lower back, the knee joints, the spinal cord, are plagued by pain and discomfort due to this adaptation. Scientists have discovered that arthritis has been a problem since hominids became bipedal. The muscular structure supports the bone structure and makes locomotion function. By strengthening the muscular frame, we can reduce the problems of pains and discomfort on the spinal cord, knees, and other structural load-carrying members. The muscle and the bones form the key load-carrying capability of the body; by making this pair of members as flexible, strong, and healthy as possible, we give the body the best chance to reduce the stress of physical nature.

Pathogens, predators, extraneous physical forces — from any source — can also be reasons for excessive stress on the body. A pathogen attacking the body can cause, for example, individual human cells to break down by breaking the protective cell membrane, and then it can create havoc on this otherwise harmonious element. Physical attack, whether from a predator, foe, or friend, can also cause severe stress if the forces are excessive. For example, a dog attack, or a car crash, or any other form of excessive load on the body, can produce fractures, body pains, and other physical complications. The sources of physical forces responsible for stress on the body are many, but by understanding the original source of the force and physical stress, one has an opportunity to eliminate this stress. In martial arts, we learn that, in order to avoid excessive stress — for example, when one is being thrown on the floor, it is necessary to "relax" the body. This relaxation makes the muscles more flexible, less rigid, which in turn translates to lower overall stress due to the act of falling. It is like breaking a glass by letting it fall on hard cement: it would break rather easily because it is very rigid. Do the same experiment and let a rubber band fall on the floor and it will never break because it is very flexible — that is the goal to obtain when searching for relaxation of the muscle and minimization of impact-driven stress.

Pain is inevitable. Suffering is optional

— Buddhist proverb

Balance—panacea to high stress

Rivers, flowing and meandering around all types of terrain, eventually end up in the oceans. The river always starts at a high area — typically on mountain peaks — and ends up at the lowest point. The difference in height between those two points is what causes a force to create the river current and movement; this is known as potential energy. A battery works in the same way, by pushing current via a wire where there is a voltage potential. When the potential disappears, the river dries or the battery dies, then the current stops. This concept of differential value at two points to create motion is universal. We can infer from this analogy that, when the system is in equilibrium, then there is no motion — no current, no flow — and if there is no motion, then there is no force or stress in the system. This concept of pressure (or stress) difference is key to understanding the physical stress of all tissues, cells, and all human body components.

Forces make the world go around. For any motion to occur, a force must be present to generate it. This is the first of Newton's law of motions, in which a force acting on a mass will cause it to accelerate. One can explain any stress on a body by the identification of the force causing it. Consider a ball rolling down a hill: the force of gravity is responsible for this motion. This view of motion helps us identify the origin of physical stress, which is similar to a physical force — remember, a force is equivalent to stress; a high force causes high stress and a low force causes small stress. In physics, one common approach to finding a force, for static systems, is to find the sum of all force and then find the balance of the system. If there is an imbalance, then there is a force or stress on the system. Applying this concept to the physical stress the human body faces, we can surmise that, if the body is in physical balance (proper alignment, good posture, good muscle mass, and proper symmetry), then the physical stress on the body will be minimal. A system in balance is one with extremely low stress. Striving for balance is equivalent to eliminating stress.

Low energy—high physical load

A body that lacks enough physical structure to support the mechanical loads imposed by the daily routines will break down often. The human body is the ultimate adaptable machine and it can change to adjust to almost any given condition. This evolutionary change, however, takes time. By maintaining the highest energy available to your capability, one will minimize the probability of body breakdowns. The main source to acquire a high level of energy and vitality is to exercise the body frequently, consistently, and with proper techniques. We will discuss exercises in future chapters, but I want to make you aware of one of the solutions to the lack of energy and vigor.

A weak body is also susceptible to attack by pathogens and foreign substances. These primarily cause chemical stress, but they can also cause physical stress by breaking down cells and tissues. These physical ruptures would cause pains, discomfort, and further body complications. The low- energy and ill-prepared physical body is a prime target for these attacks.

Strong body—minimal physical stress

The perfectly balanced body is in a state of minimum stress. A body that is aligned, erect, and correct in posture and stance is in harmony, equilibrium, and in a state of low stress. The solution to lower physical stress is to strengthen the body, building muscular structure and strength. The stronger body structure helps maintain the body erect, properly aligned, and ready to defend itself against any predators (macro or microscopic in nature).

Lack of muscular structure is one of the main drivers of physical pain. When the body lacks sufficient muscular and skeletal structure to support the normal loads, one suffers physical stress often. We see lack of structure in a humped or arched back, a bulging stomach, an arched neck, and poor posture. All of these add too much physical stress to the body, resulting in a pain signal being generated. The key to alleviating all of these is to build a muscular body with enough musculoskeletal structure to withstand all these normal daily forces and to keep the body erect and symmetric. This type of strong body is best for reducing physical stress. Athletes and high-performing individuals with well-defined and strong muscular bodies face minimum instances of maladies, and when they happen, they are short in duration.

CHAPTER 6: AND THEN THERE WERE PILLS

CHEMICAL STRESS—SYNTHETIC MALFUNCTION

In order to change, we must be sick and tired of being sick and tired.

— Unknown

O ur generation is one of the sickest we have seen in a very long time. The prevalence of chronic diseases is rampant and on the rise in the United States. According to the National Center for Chronic Diseases Prevention and Health Promotion (NCCDPHP), a chronic disease is broadly defined as a condition that lasts one year or more requires ongoing medical attention, or which limits activities of daily living, or both. Chronic diseases affect approximately 133 million Americans—40% of the population. More and more people are living with not just one chronic illness, such as diabetes, heart disease, or depression, but with two or more conditions. Six in ten Americans live with at least one chronic disease, like heart disease, stroke, cancer, or diabetes. Chronic diseases are the key drivers of the United States' $3.5 trillion annual health care cost. These conditions, sometimes called "lifestyle" diseases, are caused mostly by the environmental conditions – epigenetic changes – and the increased levels of physical, chemical, and mental stress we experience daily. A sharp increase in these factors is the main force behind these disturbing trends. Chemical stresses arise from exposure to synthetic chemicals and or environmental factors that create internal forces resulting in negative and damaging effects on the body.

Despite our advances in drug discovery and delivery, our society is today sicker than ever. Major chronic diseases are at epidemic levels in the United States. The number one killer is heart disease and stroke. More Americans die from heart disease and stroke than any other major illness. More than 860,000 die of heart disease or stroke every year. The economic impact of these on our health care system is estimated at $200 billion per year. In 2016, the latest year for which data are available, 1.7 million new cases of cancer were reported, and 598,031 people died of cancer in the United States. Cancer is the second leading cause of death in the US – one of every four deaths. More than 30 million Americans have diabetes and 1 in 4 of them do not know they have it. Diabetes can cause heart disease, kidney failure, and blindness, and the economic impact is estimated at $237 billion per year. As costly and potentially more deadly due to all its complications is obesity. Obesity affects almost 1 in 5 children and 1 in 3 adults, putting people at risk for chronic diseases such as diabetes, heart diseases, and some cancers. One in four of all Americans 17 to 24 years are too heavy to join the military. Obesity's financial impact is estimated at $147 billion per year. Alzheimer's disease is a quite common type of dementia that is also seeing a climb in occurrence. Alzheimer's disease is an irreversible, progressive brain disease that affects 5.7 million Americans. It is the sixth leading cause of death among all adults and the fifth leading cause for those aged 65 or older. In 2010, the costs were estimated at about $200 billion. By 2040, these costs are projected to jump to almost $500 billion annually.

Chemical stress—on sources and reactions

An eager youngster tells her dad, *"Dad, the tree in our backyard is dying. It is covered with black and brown spots on its leaves. What can we do?"* The wiser father heads out to assess the situation. After examining the tree very carefully, he comes back to the house with a handful of dead leaves. *"Look, my daughter,"* he said. *"The tree is cured. It has no more dead leaves!"* The daughter looks back at the tree and she sees a very healthy, bright, and beautiful tree. The problem seems to be solved; however, she is not quite convinced. The next day, she goes out again and finds the same amount of dead leaves on the tree. *"Dad, the tree is dying again!"* she screams. The dad goes through the same routine and tells her, *"See, the tree is good now."* After several weeks have gone by and she has become used to her dad's routine, she decides one day to add water to the tree. Miraculously, the brown leaves start to disappear, and after she cemented the water routine, the tree was no longer sick. This is the model of our modern medical system. Traditional doctors do not address the root cause of the problem and are content with writing a prescription to alleviate disease symptoms. This is what happens, for example, when one is given medication for type 2 diabetes, a very treatable disease that can be completely cured in a matter of months. Pills give us temporary relief, but one must continue to take them; that is why the pharmaceutical and medical industries are so profitable, and that is the reason also for the gigantic increase in the number of prescriptions. One must demand one's health care provider the real cause of one's disease and a course of action, a plan, to cure it, not just mask it.

In 1971, President Richard Nixon declared war on cancer. Nearly 60 years later, we are still fighting the war on cancer and with no end on sight. We are losing the war as the cases of cancer continue to rise and cancer is the second leading cause of death in the US. This is a very gloomy scenario, but it is the reality of the lifestyle that our modern society has decided to adopt. The sedentary lifestyle in the United States, and the overuse of stimulants and exposure to toxic substances, are the primary causes of these trends. Toxicity, as defined by Merriam-Webster "is the quality, state, or relative degree of being poisonous."

Many chemical substances slowly poison our bodies and create a state of chemical stress. The body produces and processes hundreds of thousands of chemicals, but these naturally produced substances are not toxic to the body as they have been present with us throughout our progressive evolution. It is the exposure to industrial, synthetic chemicals that is producing this state of toxicity and contributing to the high incidence of diseases now present. Nurture and nature both play a role in this increasing trend of chronic disease prevalence. Genetic science says that genetics (i.e., genes) loads the gun, but the environment (i.e., nurture) pulls the trigger. This is a reference to our state of overall health and the factors influencing it. We have looked at the physical sources of stress and reviewed how this affects our overall health state. In this section, we are going to focus on the chemical reactions that happen inside the body and that are contributing to increasing our stress level via these reactions.

The increasing trend of chronic diseases is also leading to over-prescription and the use of OTC medication to try to manage these illnesses. The increase of pill usage is directly related to the increase in the prevalence of illness, the lack of fitness, and the overall poor bodily condition. Pill overuse is also leading to an alarmingly high pace of chemical stress, driven by the side effects of these synthetic chemicals. The medical industry's reaction to this ever-increasing trend has been to prescribe more pills and procedures. This illogical process of treating the symptoms of diseases and not addressing the real causes of illness is, unfortunately, a very profitable model for the chemical industry, the medical industry, and all other associated businesses. Profit is the main motivator in the increasing trend of pills and more pills. There is a small, growing group of holistic and functional doctors who are looking to get this trend back on track and they are starting to treat the true cause (i.e., the root) of the diseases rather than just the symptoms but, unfortunately, this is a small minority.

Our immune system is our key defense against the chemical stresses generated by these overexposures. If one properly feeds the immune system, it gets stronger in spite of our abuse to the body. It continues to adapt to defend our body the best way it can. As we identify the causes of chemical stress on our lives, the solution lies in eliminating, or reducing to the minimum, our sources of chemical and toxic environmental exposures. We need to strengthen our immune system to have the highest chance against chemical stresses.

⁂

Chemical stresses arise when the source of the force is chemical in nature. The human body runs thousands of reactions during the normal course of living to maintain, keep, grow, kill, and manage the overall interactions of the trillions of cells it possesses. In our discourse, we would be mainly concerned with chemical reactions that occur due to the introduction of foreign or artificial chemicals in the body. Examples of this interaction and reaction are the ones occurring due to human interaction with the outside environment. Synthetic chemicals are the main causes of chemical stress. The foreign nature of these products heightens the level of chemical stress as opposed to the natural chemical reactions constantly occurring in the body. Most process in nature involve chemical reactions of one kind or another. All the human senses are points of input for these chemical interactions. Matter in the form of molecules (taste and touch), electromagnetic waves (vision), smog, fumes (smell), and noise (hearing) are all potential sources of stress in the human cellular structural system. Toxins found in additives, flavor enhancers, preservatives, colorant, plastics, lotions, processed food, water, perfumes, cleaners, make-up, clothing, and several other synthetics molecules are the primary sources of chemical stress.

The exposure to synthetic chemicals spiked during the industrial revolution and beyond. The Toxic Substance Control Act (TSCA) is a United States law passed by the US Congress in 1976 and administered by the US Environmental Protection Agency (EPA) which regulates the introduction of new or already existing chemicals. When TSCA was put in place, all existing chemicals were considered safe for use and as such were grandfathered in. TSCA's key objectives were to assess and regulate new commercial chemicals, to regulate chemicals already in existence (as of 1976), and to regulate the distribution and use of these chemicals. Currently, existing chemicals on the market are listed in the

TSCA Inventory. The EPA is tasked with protecting the public from dangerous and potentially carcinogenic substances. However, there are over 62,000 chemicals that were never tested by the EPA because they were grandfathered in and statutorily not considered an "unreasonable risk." There are potentially hundreds of thousands of chemicals, that were never tested for safety, to which the public is being exposed.

The effect of these substances is unknown, but one can infer that the rise in chemical stress and diseases is a result of these exposures. As of 2015, 250 of the more than 60,000 existing chemicals have been directly tested by the EPA. Many environmental groups, such as the Natural Resources Defense Council, complain that the EPA is nearly powerless to take regulatory action against dangerous chemicals, even those known to cause cancer or other serious health effects. There is a consensus that TSCA has failed to ensure chemical safety. Even though the EPA gets notifications when new chemicals are introduced, these often come with little to no safety data and the products can go on the market without any safety review or explicit EPA approval. Bureaucratic hurdles make it more difficult for the EPA to get data on chemicals presently existing in the market and even harder to regulate them. The law is so ineffective that the EPA was overruled when it attempted in 1989 to ban deadly asbestos. As documented by EWG's 2009 *Off the Books* report, one of the biggest weaknesses of the TSCA is that chemical companies have too much leeway to hide information about their products. Companies can claim that their chemicals are "trade secrets" and they do not have to share the chemicals with state or local authorities. Keeping the information secret handcuffs the EPA and the public-at-large from assessing whether these chemicals are safe. In fact, these chemicals are the main sources of chemical-related illnesses and chemical stresses.

We are constantly learning more about the side effects of exposure to some of the many toxic chemicals the medical and chemical industries continue to push on us. We are starting to test more of them, and we have been adding to the list of toxic chemicals. Let us consider BPA (Bisphenol A); a chemical used to make plastics. BPA is found in water bottles, medical devices, beverage cans (inside liners), and sports equipment, just to name a few. These chemical leaches out of the plastic into liquids and foods. The Center for Disease Control and Prevention found measurable amounts of BPA in the bodies of 93% of the US population studied. Infants and children are estimated to have the highest daily intake of BPA because they are more exposed to this chemical—in their foods and in other plastics they use. In a study of low-income and ethnically diverse pregnant women, BPA was found in the cord blood of all women, and one-third had BPA levels that have been found to be high-risk in animals. BPA was originally developed as a synthetic estrogen, and it mimics and interferes with the action of that hormone, which helps regulate development and reproduction. BPA is called an endocrine disruptor because it affects the body's own hormones in ways that could be potentially harmful. BPAs have been found to cause serious harm, such as increased risk of heart diseases, diabetes, obesity, sexual dysfunction, and behavior problems in children. A recent study suggests that we can significantly lower our level of BPA by avoiding many packaged foods and beverages, and also change how we cook and store food. One needs to find out which products one is being exposed to that contain BPA and then eliminate this use. BPA exposure is a good example of chemical-induced stress.

Another synthetic chemical to consider as a major chemical-stressor to humans is glyphosate. Glyphosate is a broad-spectrum systemic herbicide (weed killer) and crop desiccant. Glyphosate acts in plants by disrupting the shikimic acid pathway through inhibition of the enzyme 5-enolpyruvylshikimate-3-phosphate (EPSP) synthase. The deficiency in EPSP production leads to the reduction in aromatic amino acids that are vital for protein synthesis and plant growth. Glyphosate is absorbed across the leaves and stems of plants and is translocated throughout the plant. Plants exposed to glyphosate display stunted growth, loss of green coloration, leaf wrinkling, and tissue death. Death of the plant may take from 4 to 20 days. Glyphosate was discovered to be an herbicide by Monsanto (now Bayer) in 1970. Monsanto introduced it to the market in 1974 under the name Roundup. Glyphosate is one of the most widely used herbicides in the world with applications in agriculture, forestry, industrial weed control, lawn, garden, and the aquatic environment. Sites with the largest usage include soybeans, field corn, pasture, and hay. In the United States, according to the EPA, 100 million pounds are applied every year. Worldwide, an estimated 6.1 billion kilos of glyphosate-based weed killers were sprayed across gardens and fields between 2005 and 2014. That is, by far, more than any other herbicide in the world, which leads to why it is so critical to understand the impact of glyphosate on humans and on the planet's health. Researchers have also recently found that one of Roundup's inert ingredients can kill human cells, particularly embryonic, placental, and umbilical cord cells. In reference to this finding, a study from the France's University of Caen wrote: "This clearly confirms that the [inert ingredients] in Roundup formulations are not inert." The French team commented also, "Results highlight the need for health agencies to reconsider the safety of Roundup. (Yoshida, 2016)" The research team suspects that Roundup might cause pregnancy problems by interfering with hormone production, possibly leading to abnormal fetal development, low birth weight, or miscarriages. Recently, an environmental group petitioned Argentina's Supreme Court, seeking a temporary ban on glyphosate use after an Argentine scientist reported a high incidence of birth defects and cancers in people living near crop-spraying areas. Scientists there also linked genetic malformation in amphibians to glyphosate. Additionally, a scientific team in Sweden found that exposure to glyphosate is a risk factor for people developing non-Hodgkin lymphoma. In 2005, a University of Pittsburg ecologist added Roundup at the manufacturer's recommended dose to ponds filled with frog and toad tadpoles. When they returned two weeks later, they found that 50 to 100 percent of the populations of several species of tadpoles had been killed. In March 2015, the World Health Organization's International Agency for Research on Cancer (IARC) classified glyphosate as "probably carcinogenic in humans" (category 2A) based on epidemiological studies, animal studies, and *in vitro* studies. There are hundreds of studies showing that Roundup and similar weed killers are bad for one's health. One does not need to completely understand the mechanism described above to fully appreciate the negative impact of these products on the body. People that use these products daily know to cover their mouths and limit their exposure. As an educated consumer, it is one's responsibility to scan food labels, learn about its effect, and research ways to consume glyphosate-free foods. It is also important to note that glyphosate does not just exist on the exterior of the plant; it is absorbed into the plant. Glyphosate contamination cannot be eliminated by washing the food and it cannot be broken down by cooking. One needs to get rid of foods that are contaminated with glyphosate and avoid any exposures. Glyphosate exposure has risen at a rate of 500 percent since genetically modified organisms (GMO) were introduced. Education about this and several other chemical stressors is our first step to reducing and or eliminating the negative effects of these chemicals.

Phthalates are a group of industrial chemicals that are endocrine disruptors. They are chemicals that add flexibility and resilience to consumer and building products (like polyvinyl chloride (PVC) or vinyl plastics. Close to 90% of all phthalates are used in vinyl; they are used in building products and many other consumer and commercial products. Phthalate plasticizers are not chemically bound to vinyl and they can leach or migrate into one's breathing environment. Human exposure can happen through inhalation, ingestion, and other skin exposures. Phthalates are hormone-disrupting chemicals that interfere with the production of sex hormones, especially testosterone, which is needed for "maleness" and for reproduction. Animal studies have shown that phthalates are associated with infertility, decreased sperm count, penis malformations, and undescended testes. Phthalates have also been linked with obesity, reduced female fertility, low birth weight, worsening of allergy and asthma, and altered toddler behavior. A recent risk assessment by the Chronic Hazard Advisory Panel (CHAP) of the Consumer Product Safety Commission concluded that 10% of pregnant women and 5% of infants are exposed to unsafe levels of phthalates in the US

Vaccines, a biological chemical that provides active acquired immunity to a particular disease, are also additional sources of chemical stress. Vaccines are usually an agent that is similar to the disease-causing microorganism, and it is often made from a weakened or killed form of the microbe, its toxins, or one of its surface proteins. The vaccine stimulates one's immune system to recognize the agent as a threat and to prepare an attack to fight the pathogen. A memory is created in the immune system to which it can respond in case a similar attack is faced in the future, destroying the attacker. Although vaccines have helped to contain several viral diseases and are considered generally safe in the short term, there is a lot of area for concern when it comes to ingredients contained in them and the number of vaccines — over 72 vaccines for a typical child vaccine schedule — currently required. Vaccines are known to contained neurotoxin, heavy metals elements that could cross the brain barrier, and these have been linked to neurological diseases.

The body of evidence is exceptionally large and It is not my intention in this section to detail all the pros and cons of vaccines. As an educated consumer, however, I recommend one study both sides of the argument. Do not take for granted the statement that vaccines are safe, and that the government is looking out for your health and best interests. One needs to evaluate the evidence for both arguments and then make an educated, scientific conclusion. There is no doubt that vaccines cause chemical stress in the body that could result in serious and debilitating diseases like Alzheimer's, cancers, and many others. Before blindly taking a vaccine because a "white coat" recommends it, first study its components, the effects, and completely compare the risks versus the rewards of this option. Then, and only then, should you proceed. This is the Efenian way: it is acting on scientifically verifiable evidence and then making the smart choice. Question the need for the vaccine. Is it really needed at this time? What are the risks and rewards of the particular dosage in question? Additional, long term studies are needed to understand the real health effects of some of the toxins present in some vaccines. The prevalence of mental ills like autism seem to be highly correlated to the increasing use of vaccines. This is a red flag that additional scientific studies need to be done to fully understand this relationship.

AND THEN THERE WERE PILLS

Practice two things in your dealings with disease: either
help or do not harm the patient.

— Thomas Inman, MD

Pills, pills, and more pills—an industry is birthed

Medical drug (pill) prescriptions have steadily increased for the past few decades. The latest report from IQVIA Institute reported that there were 5.8 billion prescriptions dispensed in 2018, up 2.7 percent from the previous year. More than two-thirds of the total prescriptions were for chronic conditions, which are increasingly filled with 90-day prescriptions. The out-of-pocket cost for retail prescription drugs is estimated to have been $61 billion in 2018. Although this explosion of medication prescriptions in some instances save lives, the majority of these are for preventable and curable illnesses like type 2 diabetes and obesity-induced diseases. Not all these prescriptions have been beneficial to humans. A 2016 study estimated the number of deaths that were a result of medical errors in the US to be 251,000. The elders are hardest hit as the average number of prescriptions for this group is about 15 per year. Every combination of drugs increases the risk of harmful drug interaction and the possibility of complications. It is important to keep in mind that prescription medicines can be just as dangerous, when misused, as street (illegal) drugs. Prescription drugs, over-the-counter drugs, and many other industrial chemicals contained in medicine, home cleaning, and many other industrial products, are the primary sources for chemical stresses.

Natural remedies have been used as medicine for millennia. Early men used herbs, animals, trees, and many other organic materials to produce a blended version of medicines. The growth in the synthesis of medicines was catalyzed by our increase in chemical knowledge and greater rigor in using science for the blending. The alchemists started to use more scientific methods and began documenting their experiments. The introduction of synthetic heroin started in the nineteenth century. It was first thought to be non-addicting but was later found to be so addictive that health professionals, and the public institution at large, called for its ban and control. Aspirin was introduced in 1899 by the Bayer company. Aspirin was introduced into medical practice due to its perceived effectiveness; Bayer originally promoted it to doctors. This was one of the first medicine that had some positive effect and were not addictive. In 1900, opium, morphine, and cocaine came into wide use in over-the-counter medicines made by pharmacists or manufacturers, known as patent medicines. As medicines continue to flood the market, the government started to regulate its production. In 1919, the United States vs Doremus court case confirmed that the federal government could regulate the dispensing of medicines by physicians. During the prohibition of alcohol (1928), doctors were allowed to write special prescriptions for pints of whiskey or wine for their patients. Millions of prescriptions were written and dispensed. Much of this alcohol was not used for medical purposes, resulting in the greatest diversion of prescription medicines prior to the present time. By 1933, we saw the introduction of amphetamines into the United States. The military on both sides of WWII used amphetamines. It was given on both sides of the combat to assist soldiers in staying awake during long days and nights. Amphetamine use by civilians would not increase until after the war. A few years later, marijuana came under federal control. By 1938, Amendments to the Pure Food and Drug Act brought the abuse of non-narcotic medicines under the responsibility of the FDA.

A disturbing trend on the increased use of prescribed and OTC drugs is the illicit usage of these products. In the US alone, an estimated 55 million people have used prescription drugs for nonmedical reasons in their lifetime. The majority of misused drugs include painkillers, stimulants, tranquilizers, and sedatives. Prescribed drugs are as large a part of the overall drug problem as is the use of restricted drugs like marijuana, cocaine, and other hard drugs. Nonmedical use of Adderall (2006-11) and emergency visits involving drugs increased significantly: Adderall misuse rose 67 percent; ER visits went up 156 percent. Young adults (18-25 years old) made up 60 percent of those using Adderall for nonmedical reasons. The use of Benzodiazepine prescription increased 76 percent (from 8.1 to 13.5 million) between 1996 and 2013. While the total quantity prescribed more than tripled, during the same period, the overdose death rate for benzodiazepines more than quadrupled. Today, all states have prescription drug monitoring programs. Prescribed medications, OTC medications, and the illicit usage of pills are creating the chemical stress and symptoms of our very sick society. Every drug that we take, whether legal or illegal, causes chemical reactions in the body, which could potentially cause the body to break down and manifest diseases.

Side effects—by prescriptions

Although I am not of the belief that one should eliminate all of one's current medications, I do believe that it should be one's goal to eventually use neither prescribed nor OTC medications at all. Only sick people need medication; once one becomes truly healthy there is no need for them. Of course, you should work with your personal physician to ensure you do this in a safe and reasonable manner. As a person committed to total fitness, you should strive for the total elimination of any type of prescribed or OTC drugs. There is room for medications in emergencies, for chronic conditions, and or in critical or last resort scenarios. In those instances, these drugs are life-saving options. But, for most people taking pills, this is not the case. When you next visit your doctor, challenge him or her to tell you what is the "root cause" of your illness or what is it that is broken that requires you to have to take this synthetic medical intervention. If you do not get a satisfying solution, then you should fire your doctor and find one that is focused on holistic medicine and looks at the real cause of illness, not just treating a given symptom. All medicines have side effects. Avoid the use of overprescribed pills (i.e., medicines), processed food, and supplements. All the nutrients the body needs to get well and thrive can be gotten from organic, wholesome foods. Most medical doctors are very poorly trained to cure common diseases and to provide preventive care. The main system of care in today's medical industry is one of managing symptoms. The myriad of drugs in the market are driven by greedy, profit-driven pharmaceutical companies, whose main concerns are to produce a profit. You must be an educated consumer and question every diagnosis and, if in doubt, get a second opinion. In this age of easy research and information at our fingertips, there is no excuse for not being well informed on any potential medically-prescribed medications.

In addition to synthetic pills, another key source of chemical stress is the food we eat. In later chapters, we will explore the role of food on the body. Foods, through chemical reactions, aid in the support, growth, and reproduction of the body. These reactions are sources of chemical stress as well, some good for the body, others not so beneficial. At this stage, just consider the food as a potential source of chemical stress. We will detail these mechanisms further down the road.

The key to diminishing and or vanishing any chemical stress is to find its source and address its elimination and or reduction. We have identified the primary source as arising from the consumption and exposure to synthetic chemicals. By only focusing on natural exposure to chemicals and exposure only to essential synthetics (in case your body cannot produce it, or one cannot obtain it in a natural way), one will get rid of the side effects that are causing the most of our current ills. *"If man makes it, do not eat it."* This is a great rule of thumb to avoid consuming synthetic and processed chemicals that lead to chemically-induced stress.

CHAPTER 7: MENDACIOUS SYNDROMES

MENTAL STRESS—MINDFUL FLOW

All that we are is the result of what we have thought

— Buddha

T he human brain is a universe within. There are more than one hundred billion neurons—brain cells— in our brain, and each one of these has thousands of connections to each other and to other cells of the body—like the branches of a tree. These connections are a thousandth of a millimeter in size and are called synapses. There are trillions of synaptic connections in our brains, which is larger than the number of stars in our galaxy. Our brains are a miracle of nature. The pattern of all these connections is sometimes referred to as the connectome—a comprehensive map of neural connections in the brain— and may be thought of as its wiring diagram. Because every connection is said to be some type of information—data, memories, processes, learning, etc.— you are your collection of memories; you are your connectome. The complexity of our brain arises from the remarkably high number of possible states that the connections can control – estimated to be around 100 trillion connections! Homo sapiens are overly complex because we are the only animal on our planet with a highly evolved brain cerebral cortex. The cortex is the outer part of our brain, and it was the latest part to be developed during our evolutionary ladder. At the embryonic level, the first part that gets developed is our primitive brain – sometimes referred to as our mammalian brain. Our uniquely developed brain, with its cerebral cortex, gives us a unique and competitive advantage over all living species: the ability to think. This critical ability to think allows us to create tools, outsmart competitors, adapt quickly and efficiently, and in short, give us the ability to become the alpha of all currently known species. We stand today at the top of the food chain, mostly due to our unique, competitive advantages, our intelligence. Our brains use this capacity for intelligence to create an internal, optimized model to perceive the reality of the outer environment, our internal reality. When our internal models are in harmony with the environment in which they live, we are said to be in a fit mental state. Breakdowns occur when our internally-created perception conflicts with the outer reality.

These breakdowns are caused by mental stress. Mental stress occurs when the factor causing the tension on the body is mental in nature. While the bulk of mental stress is, in general, our own creation (nurture) as a result of how we see the world, another large portion of mental stress comes from genetic factors (nature). The 2018 Gallup report on the world's emotional state shows Americans were more likely to be stressed and worried than much of the rest of the world. The report found that 55% of Americans experienced stress – one of the highest rates out of the 143 countries studied, and it beat the global average (35%) by 20 percentage points. When we consider that stress is something that frequently occurs on our lifespan, then the true incidence of stress is much higher than what is being reported. Being stressed is a phenomenon that affects almost everyone. The stressor (or triggers) for mental stress are many, including daily hassles, life events, social interactions, financial concerns, and many other ongoing, long-term demands. Different people, facing the same event, experience different levels of mental stress; each one will experience the event in a unique way, based on their internal model of the world. Some people are more vulnerable than others to becoming stressed in any given situation. A simple event like dealing with a daily commute can cause severe stress on some individuals, while others barely notice this stressor. The individual reaction to stressors depends on several factors, including your mental toughness, biological makeup, perception, and ability to cope with challenges.

No one saves us but ourselves. No one can and no one may.
We ourselves must walk the path.

— Buddha

A path to mental health—stress root cause

Mental stressors are stimuli created within our brains which cause you to move to a negative state of mind, ultimately resulting in suffering and or pain. Currently, there is an avalanche of mental disorders. According to the National Institute of Mental Health, nearly one in five US adults live with a mental illness (46.6 million in 2017). Youth mental health is worsening. From 2012-17, the prevalence of past-year Major Depressive Episodes (MDE) increased from 8.66 percent to 13.01 percent. Now, over two million youth have MDE with severe impairment. When we look at cases of mental disorders—depression, dementia, Alzheimer's, ADD, bipolar, etc.—the trend is clearly moving upwards. Why, with the advent of many prescription drugs, therapies, and modern technologies, are these mental diseases still increasing? There are several theories to explain the rise in prevalence. The pace of life has increased dramatically as compared to ten years ago. The surge of the internet has changed the landscape, where most individuals spend an average of more than eight hours being exposed to electronic media of one form or another. The brain suffers from overstimulation caused by all this media fighting for one's attention. This increased demand for one's limited attention span comes with a heavy price. Those individuals that have a coping mechanism and were able to quickly adapt to additional mental stress due to the additional demands for attention, including the attacks of advertising and social media, have been able to joyfully survive; however, the vast majority have suffered the inevitable consequences: a depressed, stressed state of mind. An abundance of overstimulation has an adverse effect on a young and developing brain and adds a high level of stress to the adult (more developed brain). With no time to unplug and reconnect with friends, families, and nature, the modern Homo sapiens are getting sicker and sicker.

The fast pace of our industrial and technological societies is multiplying the sources and quantity of mental stressors. On average, Americans are living one paycheck at a time. A lack of saving discipline, combined with a culture of spending, is a key source of financial stress. Money — or rather the lack of it — is the root of most of the poor and working-class stress. When you do not have enough assets to comfortably take care of the necessities of food, shelter, and security, the body gets mentally stressed.

Another stressor, and with the strongest influence, is the one we create as a consequence of our perception of external realities. Consider the twins, Joe and Rachael: they had just lost their parents to a brutal, fatal, car crash. Joe was able to say goodbye to his parents prior to the accident; he had kept an open and loving relationship with his parents. He faced the news with maturity, reasonableness, and resolve. He managed the grief process and consequently was able to move on with his life. Rachael had many unresolved issues with her parents, and their relationship was dismal at best. She barely spoke to them and only sought them in an emergency or a must-go family situation. Rachel never had a chance to remediate her relationship with her parents. Tragically, the incident was too much for Rachel to deal with and she ended up committing suicide. How can one event affect two similar individuals (twins) in such a dramatically different way? The answer is that they each perceive the event in their own way. They each have their own mirror through which they look at life. Life itself is viewed differently, depending on which colored mirror we use. This relatively simple mechanism is the main source of most mental stress. An individual looking at life with a victim mentality, a negative outlook, a defeated attitude, will constantly be faced with mental stressors. All those stimuli will act as stressors. The body and mind are connected, and when the mind is ill (because of mental stressor), the body also gets ill. With that in mind, it should be our goal to clearly identify where is the source of mental stress is coming from and quickly and effectively deal with it. Your mental model defines your reality.

The allegory of the cave (*Plato's Cave*) was introduced by Plato in his work, Republic (514 - 520AD). It was written as a dialogue between Plato's brother, Glaucon, and his mentor Socrates: Plato has Socrates describe a group of people who have lived chained to the wall of a cave all of their lives, facing a blank wall. The people watch shadows projected on the wall from objects passing in front of a fire behind them and give names to these shadows. The shadows are the prisoner's reality. Socrates explains how the philosopher is like a prisoner who is freed from the cave and comes to understand that the shadows on the wall are not reality at all, for he can perceive the true form of reality rather than the manufactured reality that is the shadows seen by the prisoners. The inmates of this place do not even desire to leave their prison, for they know no better life. The prisoners manage to break their bonds one day and discover that their reality was not what they thought it had been. They discovered the sun, which Plato uses as an analogy for the fire that man cannot see behind. Like the fire that casts light on the walls of the cave, the human condition is forever bound to the impressions that are received through the senses. This beautiful analogy depicts how difficult it is to break away from our current reality and shines the light on what really matters to us, which is the reality that our brains create. To break from the chains of our imagined reality, one must seek an escape. The escape comes from searching for understanding. Once one understands how the stressor is having its effect on one's mind, then one can act on it. Then one starts climbing out of the cave.

Mental stressors are primarily our own creations. All humans create a mental model of the world. This model may or may not agree with reality but, regardless, your own model is what matters most to you because it is yours. The creation of mental stressors stems from the view or interpretation that this model makes of any given situation.

The mind is its own place, and in itself
Can make a Heav'n of Hell, a Hell of Heav'n.

— John Milton

The stress response—the relaxed response

On a misty morning in the middle of a Texas fall, I started my routine, early run. Being a weekend, I was to complete a half-marathon this time. These runs are my "me" times; I treasure this time and, while running, let my mind wander and engage in lively discussions with my inner self. This is the source of my creative ideas. This run took me through a vast and empty housing development area in its early stages. The area was perfect for my run as there were no cars to worry about, and the paved road, devoid of houses, provided an ideal running track. At the height of my run, out of the corner of my eye, I spotted a bulldog racing towards me. His head, disproportionately large when compared to his strong muscular body, bobbed up and down as he continued to narrow the distance between us. Sharp teeth, defiantly displayed, were smeared with saliva as he tried to cool down and reach his prey. The approaching animal made me freeze in my tracks. At this time, my entire body transformed: I felt a cold chill running all over my body, and a rush of blood filled my entire head. Time stopped to a crawl. I saw all the possibilities—as in a slow-motion movie—of this imminent dog attack, and they all included extremely bloody outcomes for both of us. After freezing for what seemed a long time (but was only a fraction of seconds), my brain decided to opt for the fight response.

The first thing I noticed was my heart beating extremely fast. Each beat was as if the heart was trying to escape my chest. My time was no longer the same as regular time. Now I had time to see every frame go by, one at a time, incredibly detailed and slow. The clarity of the actions around me seemed to be happening in a different dimension, a time-defying one. I seemingly had plenty of time to decide my course of action. I saw every step of my attacker in minute detail. I recall being amazed as to why he was taking so long to get to my area. My martial arts training took over and my muscle memory prepared my body to face the attacker. My legs sprung to an open, stable stance. I reached for the closest weapon I could find, which my mammalian brain decided was my water-carrying backpack — not sure how this was going to help — maybe by trying to put it around his mouth somehow and close his powerful teeth. My arms moved up and close to my body in a defensive pose. After unbuckling my backpack, I saw myself readying for the attack. I surveyed the whole area to search for an escape route as soon as a chance presented itself. I also quickly surmised that this would not work, as the dog would just chase me and devour me easily — the only choice was to fight. I noticed a collar on the dog, which somehow signaled to me that he might have an owner and just maybe had received some training. Although this was comforting, it did not modify my response as he continued to race toward me. With my legs quivering from the imminent battle, and with every instinct in high alert, I was resigned to the potentially deadly encounter. When the menacing dog was just a few feet away, I heard a strong voice in the background: *"Terry, stop! Come here, boy!"* An immense sigh of relief came over my body as the dog stopped and changed his direction to go back to his owner, who remained out of sight. This is the freeze-fight-flight response at work.

The brain has two distinct parts: the old brain (mammalian brain) and the new brain (cerebral cortex). They operate most of the time sequentially. We are either being driven by the mammalian brain or by the logical cerebral cortex. Our mammalian brain, designed to keep us alive, takes over in survival situations, and with utmost precision, it only gives priority to the organs and muscles needed for the response. Time is of the essence in this response. The logical brain or cerebral cortex will take too long to analyze the situation and come up with a plan of attack. The mammalian brain — sometimes called the reptilian brain — is much faster and, coupled with muscle memory, manages to keep us alive. The problem is that this brain does not distinguish between a dog's threat and a verbal threat: to the mammalian brain, it is just a threat. It goes into this kind of response whenever it feels we are under attack. This response produces cortisol, adrenaline, and other stress hormones to speed the heart and stimulate our muscles for the escape. This is an overly critical response when we are under attack, but it is not when we are just being late for a meeting, or not finding parking at the supermarket. This is the main source of mental stress for most humans. The stress response can work against you. One can turn it on when one does not really need it, as a result of a perceived emergency. It can even turn on when you are just thinking about past or future events. Harmless, chronic conditions can be intensified by the stress response activating too often, with too much intensity, or for too long.

The mind has conscious and subconscious components. At the subconscious level, one has extraordinarily little control of the mind — even though, some masters can even affect this level. Our brain also reacts through reflex loops to outside stimuli, and we have little control of this reaction. The stress response, the fight or flight response, falls in this category. The stress response is the emergency reaction system of the body. This response evolved over millions of years to keep one safe from dangers. When the stress response is turned on because the brain is perceiving some kind of threat, the body releases hormones, like adrenaline and cortisol, which signal the body to start the fight or flight response. All the organs are programmed to respond in certain ways to situations that are viewed as challenging or threatening. Without this mechanism, no animal can survive. Survival of the fittest demands this response to preserve the species for future generations.

The nervous system in charge of the stress response is called the sympathetic nervous system. The opposite response to the stress response is the "relax response." One can learn to minimize the negative stress response by learning to relax your body, by meditation, exercising, and proper nutrition. By minimizing stressful thinking, one can help the body's natural relaxation system to be amazingly effective. Your thoughts create your reality. When we practice positive thinking and have a bright outlook, our stress level is thus reduced.

Top Ten Mental Stressor Elimination Techniques

1. **Meditation**: By practicing this technique, one gives the mind a chance to reboot, and the added oxygenation aids in the formation of new brain cells (neurogenesis).
2. **Exercise**: By engaging in physical activities, one is providing an additional flow of blood to all parts of the body, thus bringing life-giving oxygen to all cells of the body. Exercise also promotes the formation of muscle, tissues, and the establishment of an optimum metabolic rate.
3. **Nutrition**: By providing proper nutrients to the brain, one is giving it the best fuel to perform optimally. Proper brain nutrition means a toxic-free regimen of food that is wholesome and natural.
4. **Rest**: Resting and proper sleep aid the brain by giving it time to rewire itself and to form strong neural connections critical to brain functions.
5. **Cultivate the Relaxation Response**: One should avoid situations where the body is in the stress response for any long period of time. By training to be in the relaxation response, one will counter the effects of the stress response.
6. **Positive Outlook**: A realistic, optimistic approach to life fine-tunes our internal model of reality and increases the chances of favorable outcomes in all one's endeavors.
7. **Mindful Living**: One should live in the present and learn to appreciate every moment, all the time, creating a happy life and a content mind.
8. **Purposeful Living**: Finding a life purpose gives direction to our actions, and this force promotes the creative brain. Not having a purpose is akin to being in a boat in the middle of the ocean, without any idea of where one wants to go.

9. **Engage in "Flow" Activities**: These are activities where one is "in the zone." In flow, we lose the concept of time, and one is fully immersed in the act and will it do forever, if possible. These activities keep the brain fit and stress-free.

10. **Create a Personal Vision**: A personal vision, with specificity on your goals, keeps the mind grounded, and provides the fuel to perform daily at a high level.

Execution Begets Peak Performance

Live as if you were to die tomorrow. Learn as if you were to live forever.

— Mahatma Gandhi

E xecution — the art of getting things done — eludes us all. Many plans and brilliant ideas die on the vine because creators lack the fortitude to execute, to follow through on their vision. What differentiates those that can get things done efficiently and consistently and those who do not is all in the execution of their plan. What makes someone like Christopher Columbus cross an unknown ocean without truly knowing his destination? What makes a dreamer wake up with the conviction that today will be their day? What makes people do what they must when they should? It is the desire to make things that matter happen, the desire and will to do, to execute!

Excuses abound: There is no lack of words and or stories to find a reason why not to execute. It comes naturally to languorous minds as it is the state of lowest energy. To do nothing requires no energy. To spend energy on what we find worthwhile is divine and, paradoxically, by spending the energy, we get rewarded with more energy in return. When deciding on a specific action to do, it is helpful to answer this question: What is the *"possibility for action"*? Every action has a reaction. Is the reaction to what I am about to do worth the execution? Is it a positive reaction? If the answer is no, then do not do it. This tool can be applied to any controversial or difficult decision one needs to make. To apply it, simply ask yourself, what is the possibility for action of what I am about to do or say? An honest answer to this question will, one hundred percent of the time, yield a positive outcome in any situation.

When one thinks of a character that can execute, get the work one, accomplish and follow through on his vision, the name Mahatma Gandhi jumps to mind. If we call execution the art of doing, then Gandhi was the painter of its canvas. In India, he was named Mahatma, "Great Soul." Gandhi was the most prominent leader of the Indian Independence movement, and, in India, he is unofficially referred to as "Father of the Nation." Even more incredible is that he accomplished all this through non-violence movements. He was always getting things done, stirring emotions, organizing rallies, protesting and resisting, and propagating ideas that would ultimately create a passive revolution. Gandhi was responsible for the creation of a nation, India. He started his activism while being an immigrant in South Africa, in the early 1900s, and became the face of India's struggle for independence from Great Britain.

In 1869, Gandhi was born into an Indian Gujarati Hindu Modh Baniya family, in Porbandar, a coastal town on the Kathiawar Peninsula, the capital of the small principality in western India under British suzerainty. He was the youngest child of his father's fourth wife. His father — Karamchand Uttamchand Gandhi — was chief minister of Porbandar State. Although he did not have much formal education, Karamchand was a capable administrator who knew his way around the headstrong British officers in power. Young Gandhi was described by his sister Raliat as "restless as mercury, either playing or roaming about. One of his favorite pastimes was twisting dog's ears." Stories of the Indian classics—like stories of Shravana and king Harishchandra—impacted him very profoundly. Gandhi wrote later, in his autobiography, referring to these stories: "It haunted me, and I must have acted Harishchandra to myself times without number." His early self-identification with truth and love as supreme values are traceable to this classic character. Gandhi's mother, Putlibai, was from the medieval Krishna bhakti-based Pranami whose tradition is believed to include the essence of the Vedas, the Koran, and the Bible. She was a very pious lady who would never think of eating her meals without saying her daily prayers. She would take the hardest vows and keep them without flinching. She believed strongly in nonviolence and in that everything in the universe is eternal. Putlibai was very absorbed with religion. She did not care much for material things and divided her time between her home and the temple. She would do two or three days of fasts as if it were nothing. Gandhi was deeply influenced by his mother.

Teen Gandhi studied at the Rajkot High School, where he was an average student, won a few prizes, but was considered a shy and timid student with little interest in games—his love was books and school lessons. While in school he met his friend, Sheikh Mehtab, who encouraged him to eat meat to gain height—Gandhi was a vegetarian at the time. One day, Sheikh took young Gandhi to a brothel. Gandhi found himself lost in this house of vice and refused advances by the prostitutes of the establishment; they were both instantly sent out of the brothel. This experience caused him tremendous mental anguish and, soon after, he parted ways with his friend. He loved to go out on long solitary walks, and when in the house, would spend time helping his mother do house chores. As was customary at the time, he was betrothed to his childhood friend, Kasturbai Makhanji Kapadia. At the age of 13, he was married to the 14-year-old Kasturbai. Of his marriage day, he would later say, "As we did not know much about marriage, for us it meant only wearing new clothes, eating sweets and playing with relatives." They spend a great deal of time apart from each other and, as a result of her age, she ended up spending much time at her parent's house. In 1885, Gandhi and Kasturbai had their first child, who would survive only a few days.

During this same time, Gandhi's father passed away. Both events devastated him. Eventually, Gandhi and Kasturbai went on to have four more children.

⁓

Gandhi's family was not wealthy; he struggled to afford the cost of schools. He wanted to become a doctor; however, if he was to keep the family tradition of holding high office, he needed to study law. A priest and family friend advised him and his family that he should go to London to become a lawyer. His mother was uncomfortable with him leaving them. To convince her, Gandhi vowed to her that he would abstain from meat, alcohol, and women. Putibai gave him permission and blessings to go to London and pursue his studies. Gandhi dedicated himself to his studies while in England, but his main concerns during the three years he was there would be moral issues. He struggled constantly to try to adapt to the lifestyle of the university, as well as to Western food, dress, and etiquette. In a meat-loving society, his vegetarianism was viewed as out-of-place or outdated. His friends would warn him that his food preferences would damage his studies as well as his health. He stuck to his guns and ended up joining a vegetarian society — where he became a member of the executive committee — and these activities would fill him with confidence and help him cope with his then-current predicaments. In 1893, he headed to South Africa to work as a lawyer for a family member. He spent 21 years in South Africa, where he would mature his political and ethical views. He faced several instances of discrimination while in Africa because of the color of his skin and heritage. In one instance, he would not be allowed to sit with European passengers and was told to sit on the floor, then was beaten when he refused. In another incident, he was kicked off the footpath and onto the street without warning by a police officer — Indians were not allowed to walk on public footpaths. In South Africa, he considered himself "a Briton first, and an Indian second". However, the incidents and prejudice he saw and experienced against his fellow Indians in Africa deeply bothered him. Gandhi began to ponder his people's standing in the British Empire.

He was not extremely interested in politics; however, after suffering from several injustices, his thinking and focus changed, and he resolved to resist and fight for his and other victims' rights. People would spit on him as an expression of racial hate. He entered politics by forming the Natal Indian Congress. Gandhi and his colleagues would later help Africans as nurses and by opposing racial discrimination — according to Noble Peace Prize winner Nelson Mandela. Gandhi's stories in Africa, although not free of controversial and inconvenient truths, is mostly filled with co-operation and effort with nonwhite Africans, to help rid local Indians and Africans of persecution and apartheid. In 1906, when the Transvaal government passed an ordinance requiring all Indians to register, Gandhi headed a campaign of civil disobedience which would last for over eight years. Hundreds of Indians were arrested as a result of the protests, and thousands of Indian miners were flogged, imprisoned, and even shot. The persistent pains of this campaign — assisted by pressures from the British and Indian governments — finally forced the South African government to accept a compromise which included key concessions like the recognition of Indian marriages and the abolition of the existing poll tax for Indians.

༚

In 1914, Gandhi returned to India. He was openly critical of colonial authorities and felt their dealings were unjust. He organized a passive resistance campaign in response to Parliament's passage of the Rowlatt Act. This Act gave colonial authorities emergency powers to arrest and detain without judicial review, and to treat civil disobedience as criminal actions. After violence broke out — including the British-led massacre of more than 400 Indian protestors — Gandhi slowed down the efforts. However, he would later continue to incite nonviolent rallies and, by 1920, he was the face of the Indian movement for independence. His messages would stress the importance of nonviolent, non-cooperation campaign for home rule, and the economic independence for India. Gandhi was revered by his followers, due in great part to his eloquent style, based on prayer, fasting, and meditation.

Working with the Indian National Congress (INC), Gandhi turned the independence movement into a force to reckon with. They organized boycotts of British manufactures and of British institutions like schools and legislatures. In 1922, British authorities arrested Gandhi and tried him for sedition – he was sentenced to six years in prison but was released in 1924 after an attack of appendicitis. By 1931, the British authorities had made some concessions and Gandhi called off the resistance movement and agreed to represent the Congress Party at the Round Table Conference in London. Some of the party members were not in agreement with Gandhi's negotiation style and they were getting frustrated with, in their belief, his lack of concrete gains. One member was Mohammed Ali Jinnah – the leading voice for India's minority Muslims. Upon his return, Gandhi was arrested once more, this time by a newly aggressive colonial government. Gandhi began a series of hunger strikes to protest the treatment of India's poor classes, whom he renamed Harijans, or "Children of God." The fasting appeared to work, and it resulted in swift reforms by the Hindu community and the government. After a brief departure from politics to focus on community service, Gandhi returned to lead the INC after the onset of World War II. He demanded the British withdrawal from India in return for Indian cooperation with the war effort. British authorities, instead, imprisoned the entire INC leadership, thus bringing the relations to the lowest point ever. In 1947, the Labor Party took power in Britain. Negotiations started again between the British, the Congress Party, and the Muslin League – led by Jinnah. After the negotiations, Britain granted India its independence, but they split the country into two, India and Pakistan. Gandhi opposed the split but agreed, in the hope that after independence the Hindus and Muslims could achieve peace and reconciliation.

On January 30, 1948, Gandhi was on his way to an evening prayer meeting in Delhi when he was shot to death by Nathuram Godse – a Hindu fanatic enraged by Gandhi's efforts to negotiate with Jinnah and other Muslims. Over 1 million people attended the procession as Gandhi's body was paraded through the streets of the city and cremated on the banks of the holy Jumna River.

CHAPTER 8: MARATHON FOR EVERYONE

LIFE — A PEAK PERFORMANCE AFFAIR

Having a vision for what you want is not enough. Vision without execution is hallucination.

—Thomas A. Edison

B reathing so hard that he felt his heart was about to come out of his chest, but not minding pains, oblivious to anything else on his path, with every leg muscle torn and swollen from prior days of running, and on the final miles of his life, this runner had only one thing in mind: to convey his message of victory; and after he did, he collapsed and died. Legend has it that Pheidippides, a Greek herald in 490 B.C., was sent running from Marathon to Athens, Greece, to announce that the Athenian army had defeated the invading Persian army in a battle on the plain of Marathon, located roughly 26 miles north of Athens. Pheidippides ran in the late summer heat, and after reaching the Athenian, he is said to have exclaimed, "Nike! ("Victory!") or "Rejoice!

We Conquer," and then he collapsed dead from exhaustion. This story is the inspiration for one of the most popular sports of ultimate endurance and persistence, the marathon – a 26.2-mile race. This story was popularized in the 19th century. In 1834, French sculptor, Jean-Pierre Cortot, completed a sculpture in Paris's Tuileries Palace, of Pheidippides dying as he announced victory. In 1879, English poet Robert Browning wrote the poem "Pheidippides."

"Unforeseeing one! Yes, he fought on the Marathon day:

So, when Persia was dust, all cried 'To Akropolis!

Run, Pheidippides, one race more! the meed is thy due!

"Athens is saved, thank Pan," go shout!'

He flung down his shield, Ran like fire once

more: and the space 'twixt the Fennel-field

And Athens was stubble again, a field which a fire runs through,

Till in he broke: 'Rejoice, we conquer!' Like wine thro' clay,

Joy in his blood bursting his heart, he died – the bliss!"

Twenty years after the poem, the Marathon race was created for the 1896 Olympics. The first modern game organizers wanted to celebrate the victory of Marathon. French historian Michel Breal suggested a long-distance race from Marathon to Athens to honor Pheidippides' run, and the modern marathon was born. The Marathon has become a test of endurance and performance for runners of all ages – people, in general, aiming to get in peak physical shape. When I decided to run my first Marathon, I was fifty pounds overweight. My motivation for running was to lose excess weight and get in good physical shape. The journey to this run was very inspiring but the results I got out of the training and execution of my first Marathon were much more than I expected. The weight loss was one of the minor benefits. I was pre-diabetic, with high blood pressure, often tired and with frequent low levels of energy, had ulcers and experienced constant allergies due to pollen and several other allergens. As if by magic, after I completed my Marathon training — and finished my race — all the above ills went away. I pushed through my marathon race with the healthiest body I had ever possessed to that point. The body is self-healing and self-regulating. As I increased the demands on my physical performance of the body, the body responded by becoming better, by getting stronger, and by improving immune system performance. These benefits were one hundred times better than any pills I could take for any of my symptoms. I learned to love running, and I have made it part of my weekly routines. I came to understand what runners called the runner's high — a state of euphoria as a result of the act of running. To properly train and complete a Marathon, discipline, consistency, execution, great physical condition, and a very strong mental toughness are all needed. All these are properties of executing high performances.

Athletic performance is the mark modern society uses to measure high performance. A high-performance athlete is paid more today than any president of any country, including that of the United States of America. Why is athletic performance valued so highly? One can postulate it is our spirit of competition, our ability to win over any other thing, our desire to matter, our desire to be number one, and other similar arguments. No matter what the individual thinks the reason for the athlete's obsession is, we can all agree that the top athletes are *peak performers*. When they find themselves at their peak, they are functioning at their optimum self. This analogy can be easily expanded to all affairs of living. Top producers in business are workers that are at their peak performance. All other professions and aspects of existence are touched by operating at peak performance. It is in our nature, imprinted by evolution on our DNA, to be optimized, to operate at the highest level available to us. This produces the best version of you and the best environment for growth and happiness.

Why, then, is mediocrity and lack of performance so prevalent in our society? Mediocrity is a product of our social environment, where the natural functions required for living in a natural environment are substituted by artificial ones. The excess of "stuff" allows us to live in a quasi-comfort which does not require us to do all the necessities of body performance. Just as high physical performance is paramount to overall happiness, so is high mental performing. An individual executing at high mental capacity is one who is grounded in their thoughts and daily decisions. Their thinking is clear, with purpose, and mindfulness. Peak performance living is executing daily at your highest possible potential. We can all do a lot more than we think we can. The key is to continue to push yourself to become the best you can be in all areas.

Execution, the art of getting things done!

Execution in business was brilliantly described by Larry Bossidy and Ram Charan in their book, *The Discipline of Getting Things Done*. They argue that execution is a discipline, a process, a systematic way of exposing reality and acting on it. They explained that it is of paramount importance that a business leader knows how to execute well. One must always be asking how and what—one must ask questions and be accountable. One must be able to understand the business environment and the organization's capability. Part of executing, they argue, means having the business leader master three key roles: selecting the right people, setting the strategic direction, and coordinating operations. Execution needs to be a core part of the company culture; it needs to be the norm, with all employees on board. On an individual level, execution is similar to business execution. Instead of a business, one has one's daily tasks, one's functions, one's social responsibilities, and one's daily chores. Individual execution is required for getting things done, for performing at peak levels. Your execution level is driven by your individual goals and strategies. When a person has clear and specific personal goals and vision, they have opened the possibility for high-level execution. Without a clear direction, a sailing ship will just meander in the middle of the ocean. When there is a void of direction, there is no room or need for execution. Living becomes a mere reaction to the external environment stimulus and forces that push you around your circle of influence. When people master the art of getting things done, they learn to compete not with others but with themselves. Only then do they aim to be better every day and every second; therefore, they cannot help but execute.

Michael Jordan, one of the most successful athletes of this century, considered by most as the greatest basketball player of all time, suffered several failures throughout his career. In 1978, Jordan tried out for the varsity team at Laney High School. He was rejected. Instead, he was asked to play on the junior varsity team. The coach told him he did not have enough talent and he had not distinguished himself as an outstanding basketball player. It was not an illogical decision at the time, as the coach knew that as a junior player Jordan would get more playing time and give more opportunity to prove himself. But the 15-year old was devastated and, in his mind, this was a dismal failure. Jordan was heartbroken and ready to give up the sport until his mother convinced otherwise. After putting everything into perspective, Jordan set out to prove himself. He picked up the pieces, started working really hard and executing at the highest level. "Whenever I was working out and got tired and figured I ought to stop, I'd close my eyes and see that list in the locker room without my name on it, and that usually got me going again." For most people, failures will stop them in their tracks; Jordan used it as fuel to move forward. This will become a hallmark of his career. He would later reflect on his failures:

I have missed more than 9,000 shots in my career. I have lost almost 300 games. On 26 occasions I have been entrusted to take the game-winning shot, and I missed. I have failed over and over and over again in my life. And that is why I succeed."

— Michael Jordan

Execution is a process; it is not a one-time event. Jordan's persistence, his willingness to succeed no matter the obstacle, and his relentless drive are all levers of high-performance execution. Happiness resides in this moment of the highest level of execution. The average person has a heavyweight pulling them down, and execution does not come naturally to them. In order to master the art of execution, they must have a drive, a passion, for doing whatever task is needed to excel. Execution creates motion in a positive direction to accomplish one's goal. High performers are notorious for raising their standards along with their goals. Why just become a nurse when you can become a doctor? Why just be a good father when you can be the best dad? This highest standard is a hallmark of high performers. They do not settle for just being average; they are constantly raising the bar. This process creates excellence. Your current body reflects your standard. If you do not have the body you desire — muscular, healthy, and in the best shape it can possibly be — then you have not raised your standard high enough. This continuous improvement is the process of execution.

What we can control is our performance and our execution,
and that's what we're going to focus on.

— Bill Belichick

Execution is the fundamental tool for every successful individual. The idea of executing something or following through with your thoughts and planned actions is the key differentiator between the individual that gets things done and the one who does not. Many create the most wonderful and detailed plans of what they hope to do, but that is as far as it goes — a great plan; those plans never get executed. Leaders are those that execute well, often, and with mindful precision and determination.

Our search for enlightenment and for the best version of you can only be obtained by "executing," by getting things done! You must now be one hundred percent committed to execution. As an Efenian — a person that executes all the time — you must be a person of action. Now you are the one who does what he says he is going to do: you produce an outcome, you execute.

Athletic-like performance—everyone can

We all are in awe when our favorite athlete performs tasks that appear to be impossible for the average person to do. We live through their performance and vicariously see ourselves in the game doing this feat of performance. Most admire the athleticism but feel inside as though this is something they cannot possibly do. But athletic performance is within our reach. If our desire is to truly obtain the highest level of performance that our body can produce, if this is truly a passionate goal, then we can obtain it. This level of high performance is not out of reach. There are daily examples of high performance by highly motivated people. We see the athletic type of performance in blue and white-collar workers, painters, chefs, and all sorts of walks of life, where the individual is motivated enough.

Athletic performance is about the efforts made by an athlete to obtain very specific performance. This performance is within reach of anyone who truly desires it and does the necessary work to obtain it. The key is to be passionate about what one is searching for; this makes the journey a lot more enjoyable and the task will not feel like doing work. High performing athletes train with a purpose and with a vision that they will execute when time demands it. This not only creates a driven desire and a body that can perform, but they have trained the mind, as well, to be tough and focused. When we think, train, and work with the fervor of athletes, we also perform our daily routines like them: we excel. Performing daily at your peak, at an athletic level, is within your reach if you desire it.

"Winning is not a sometimes thing; It is an all the time thing. You do not win once in a while; you do not do things right once in a while; you do them right all of the time. Winning is a habit. Unfortunately, so is losing."

—Coach Vincent T. Lombardi

Winning is a habit—cultivate it

To win in a sport is simple in definition: it is merely to get the highest score. In life, however, to win is very subjective and it depends very much on the person considering the winning. To win, the person may get his way in an argument, for example, or, for the same event, winning may mean finding a compromise between the parties involved. These are two completely opposite definitions of winning, for the same event. One must be clear on what winning means to oneself. In any definition, however, winning is habitual and predictable. Those who cultivate the art of winning find themselves winning frequently and with ease. Mediocrity is not an option when one is in the habit of winning. When facing interaction, "winning" means to create win-win situations.

Steven Covey explains, in his book, *The 7 Habits of Highly Effective People,* that, in order to create effective interdependent relationships, one must commit to creating win-win situations that are mutually beneficial and equitable to all parties. Additionally, he states that a very key factor is keeping an abundance mentality, or the idea that there is plenty for everyone. The opposite, a scarcity mentality, means people who act as though as everything is a zero-sum game. These people have difficulty sharing recognition and find it very difficult to be happy for others' successes. When we cultivate winning, when we make it a part of our daily life, then we get on the road of high performance.

Winning is not about beating others; it is about uplifting you. In competitive situations, like sports, our main objective is to win by beating your opposition, smashing them to submission. After you have won the contest, or situation, or the event, the euphoria of the winning moment is

114

very short-lived, and within a relatively small time period we are back to our original state. It is a fleeting, minuscule emotion that lasts only the celebration time. But when you rethink winning as giving and executing at your highest you — the best version of you — the performance could not have been any better. The feeling never goes away because you know you gave it your absolute best. That is winning, and to pursue winning is to chase the highest form of you, mentally and physically. Consequently, sometimes others will say you lost the contest, but you can still be a winner — if inside of you, that was the best performance you could have done.

Natural selection favors peak performance

Nature is the ultimate optimizer. Every living organism has been shaped by natural evolution to perform at its highest level for its environment. As the environment changes, so does the organism, in a way as to maximize its ability to survive and reproduce. Humans are no exception. Nature takes millions of years to produce some of these optimized changes. Take the design of an egg, for example. An egg is the ideal shape to hold the maximum amount of life-giving fluid and at the same time is also an ideal shape to give birth because it possesses the gentlest shape that can go through the birth channel without hurting the mother. The egg surface is not too hard, not too soft, just strong enough to hold its precious cargo until the animal is ready to break through to experience life. If we live in sync with nature, we then experience this level of optimization. Living in concert with nature means eating natural food, to keep the body in its optimal physical and mental condition. When one is attuned to the natural cycles and the natural environment, the levels of artificially-created stresses are reduced to almost nothing. Consider the monk living in a monastery, consuming the most wholesome plant-based food, breathing the less-contaminated air, and working to obtain peace of mind and tranquility. This is a nature-tuned individual. I am not suggesting that we all should become monks, but while we continue to live in a modern environment, mimicking their lifestyle would be the next best thing, and would result in us obtaining our best state.

Nature endowed Homo sapiens with the largest brain in the animal kingdom. Large brains are the defining characteristics of our species. Our relatively large brain gave us intelligence and the ability to dominate all living organisms. Intelligence reigns supreme among all the traits necessary to thrive on our planet. It is our ultimate competitive advantage. But how do we come to have such relatively large brains? Our ancient ancestor, named Lucy, *by their discoveries in reference to the Beatles song "Lucy in the Sky with Diamonds,"*[lived around 4 million years ago, and the fossil was named Australopithecus afarensis. This fossil is considered to be the missing link, with a body in the realm between modern humans and animals. Its bones are like ours and it stood upright, as opposed to its quadruped ancestors. A. Afarensis brain was tiny in comparison to today's Home sapiens, nearly a third of the size. A very fundamental question in science has been, how did Lucy's relatively small brain size evolve into the Homo sapiens brain, which is three times bigger? How and why did nature produce such a large brain and unmatched intelligence? Our mental peak performance is due to our brain's ability to reason, imagine, solve problems, and in general, to think intelligently. The brain is the most complicated organ in the universe. When we consider that we have hundreds of billions of neurons, and each has thousands of connections, making the number of synapses in the trillions, then we can begin to understand the brain's complexity. Evolutionary anthropologists have suggested three broad categories of explanation as to why the human brain grew so large. They are:

- **Environmental:** Physical challenges—like finding, hunting, or remembering sources of food—provided selection pressure for bigger brains.
- **Social:** Interacting with others—either cooperatively or competitively—favored people with brains large enough to anticipate the actions of others.

- **Cultural:** People who were able to hold on to accumulated knowledge and teach it to others were most likely to reproduce. (One of these cultural factors could have been cooking. As biological anthropologist Richard Wrangham famously argued, in his 2009 book *Catching Fire*, when we learned to cook food, we got access to more easily digestible calories, which freed up energy and time to develop bigger brains.)

It is possible that a combination of all the above three factors is also a mechanism for our large brain. Natural selection favors optimization and the transformational forces experienced by our ancestors lead to the development of the high-performance brain we currently own. Our modern brains consume about twenty-five percent of all our body's metabolic energy. This is very taxing on our bodies, but it reflects the priority and primal importance of our brains. The environment plays a big role — perhaps much larger than the social factor. The environment that we provide our brain greatly affects brain performance. To maintain our high level of performance, we must constantly check what we are being exposed to, what toxic or other environmental factors could be affecting our brain and its capabilities. We should aim to eliminate all these negative components, be aware of their existence and research ways to minimize or eliminate them. The answer as to how we evolved such large brains may not be completely solved as it is hard to disentangle all the factors involved. However, we feel the brain expanded under specific evolutionary conditions. These conditions we look to emulate to keep our brain evolving and to maintain it at its highest performance level.

We are what we repeatedly do. Excellence then is not an act but a habit.

— Aristotle

Mental excellence—a product of wisdom

Mental optimum performance is mind mastery and wisdom. To perform at one's maximum mental potential means to be able to think with clarity, analytically, and with speed and precision. The road to optimum performance of mind entails processing enough wisdom to be able to reason through every mentally stressful situation. Just like one trains the body to perform, the brain can be trained as well. The brain is extremely adaptable. Neuroplasticity refers to the ability of the brain to adapt to the myriad of situations we encounter in our daily interactions. When we exercise the brain, we grow our neural networks and strengthen connections and functioning. If we are clear of mind, with a healthy mental disposition, then we can think ourselves out of the most precarious situations.

One key component of mental performance is wisdom. To gain wisdom, one must engage in all types of scientific inquiry. One needs to seek this knowledge daily, apply it to solve real problems and be consistent with this training routine. If we learn to love this process, then this practice is made a lot easier to perform and excel. By reading, arguing, practicing, and doing scientific argumentation and or mental practice, we work out our brain and prime it for wisdom and clear thinking. To be at the top of the mental ladder, we should perform better than the average individual. Our brain has to be in top condition and free of stress and illness. To maintain this high level of performance one needs to:

1. **Train your brain.** Challenge yourself daily. One can learn a new language, learn a new craft, take a new course, and so on. Breaking your regular routine also exercises the

brain, as it forces you to come up with alternative solutions to the same old problems. Take a different route to work; use your left hand for a task you normally would do with your right hand. These challenges are brain workouts.

2. **Feed your brain**. Provide your body and your brain with food that is nutritious and devoid of artificial substances and toxins.

3. **Meditation**. Meditation is a time when the brain gets to rest and rewire itself. This quiet time allows for detoxifying your mind and bringing it to positive and inspiring thoughts. Proper rest, sleeping the necessary amount, goes hand in hand with meditation. The body needs the rest to be able to heal.

4. **Avoid toxins** like excessive alcohol, cigarettes, drugs, processed food, and all other types of neurotoxins. One must be aware of how these neurotoxins are given to us in vaccines, food, and countless other chemical substances (like cleaners).

5. **Practice self-love**. One must be kind to oneself first, and then one can extend this kindness to others. When we do not love ourselves, we do not take care of our body and mind, and we suffer. Start with yourself: make this change and the optimum mental capacity will follow.

6. **Laugh frequently and often!** Laughter has been found to be healing to our body and mind. Laughter releases stress and puts our mind in a state of growth and repair.

7. **Have fun.** Just because we search for wisdom and self-mastery does not mean we stop having fun. Doing an activity that brings us pleasure, like learning to play an

instrument, reading a fun book, or learning to garden, are all activities that promote a rounded individual and they complement all areas of living. Learn to manage stress and to reduce and or eliminate it completely.

8. **Hydrate properly.** Water is the fluid that makes life as we know it possible. We need to drink enough water daily to keep all cells in our bodies functioning properly. The amount of water depends on your level of activity, but at least half a gallon daily.

9. **Exercising** regularly promotes blood flow and improves brain cognitive abilities.

10. **Build a network.** We are networks, social networks, neural-networks, friend networks, and so on. By nurturing and building these networks, we make our brain connections stronger and plentiful. This, in turn, promotes optimal brain functioning.

CHAPTER 9: A DAY ON CLOUD NINE

HAPPINESS—REDEFINED

Happiness does not depend on what you have or who you are.

It solely relies on what you think.

—Buddha

According to the World Happiness Report 2019, the happiest country in the world is Finland. The report ranks countries on six key variables that support well-being: income, freedom, trust, healthy life expectancy, social support, and generosity. The report ranks 156 countries by how happy their citizens perceive themselves to be. Finland has a low level of crime and poverty, a great health care system, and one of the best educational systems in the world. The Finns focus on balancing work-life: there are 36 holidays per year and a guaranteed position if you leave your job for a brief time and decide to come back. University is free and, if students want a loan, the interest rate is only one percent. Their government is one of the least corrupt in the world, and there are plenty of opportunities to relax on their beautiful lands.

Happiness is exceedingly difficult to measure as the most-used indexes are based on subjective measures. However, on average, the World Happiness Report is a good metric for overall country happiness and Finland does seem to have the happiest individuals. Individual happiness is defined by Merriam-Webster as being in a state of well-being and contentment. However, psychologists, philosophers, and even economists have long sought to accurately define it. A branch of psychology since the 1990s, positive psychology has been dedicated to better define and measure happiness. Positive psychology argues that happiness is a state of well-being that encompasses living a good life, one with a sense of meaning and deep contentment. Positive psychology examines what gives our lives meaning and purpose. In contrast to traditional psychology, which focuses on dysfunction and how to treat it, positive psychology explores how ordinary people can become happier and more fulfilled. According to Christopher Peterson, a pioneering researcher in the field, the positive psychology movement is founded on three maxims: *"What is good in life is as genuine as what is bad. What is good in life is not simply the absence of what is problematic. And third, the good life requires its own explanation, not simply a theory of disorder stood sideways or flipped on its head."* While these are very wide and encompassing definition of happiness, we will look to expand and redefine these parameters to include the "balance" of total living. Happiness is about balancing challenges and opportunities in all aspects of life, to create a well-rounded individual fully connected to their environment and to humanity and optimized to perform at their highest possible level.

Wisdom and the eternal search for knowledge play a key role in happiness. Being a learner and applying the acquired knowledge to fully understand happiness allows one to get closer to this state. Happiness is not a moment in time; one goes in and out of happiness; hence, the better metric to evaluate happiness is one that is more about lifestyle than it is about a single, one-time event. We need to evaluate happiness over the span of the lifetime of the individual to truly access their level of happiness. The aggregation of all those happy moments is the best metric for happiness. We all have our own personal definition of happiness, but there are ten key areas that are all-inclusive and mastering these most likely ensures the person is on a happiness flow. We will review each of the factors as we look further into what makes each one of us happier and more content.

One event in life that helps us see clearly what the happiness factors are is the realization that human life is very finite — in fact, just a blink in the immensity of our 14.5 billion years of evolution. With an average life span of about 80 years, most of us spend a very short time on this planet. When we are faced this fact and realize that the time we have left is actually very short, we suddenly realize what really matters in life: the family, true friends, wisdom, living in the present, and sense of humanity and social networks. At this point, we start to understand why being the best version of ourselves is one of the most important things we must spend time on, as there is no time for the opposite.

Harvard Medical School has one of the longest-running studies on adult development and happiness, The Grant Study. This is a 75-year longitudinal study of 268 Harvard college sophomores from the classes of 1939-1944. It has been conducted in conjunction with a study called "The Glueck Study," which is of 456 disadvantaged, non-delinquent inner-city youths who grew up in Boston during the same period. The subjects were all male and American nationality. The study is continuing to this day. The men have been evaluated every two years. Information has been gathered about their mental, physical health, career enjoyment, retirement experience, and marital quality. The study is quite unique because of its long-time span. The sample population of this study is not randomized, and the homogeneity of the study makes its results extremely specific to the type of samples used (i.e., Harvard's graduates). With these considerations in mind, we can review the inference of this study and put its result in perspective using this fact.

According to Robert Waldinger, director of the study: "The clearest message that we get from this 75-year study is this: Good relationships keep us happier and healthier." He added, "Taking care of your body is important, but tending to your relationships is a form of self-care too. That, I think, is the revelation." The Harvard scientists have concluded that "it is not how much is in your 401(k). Not how many conferences you spoke at—or keynoted. Not how many blog posts you wrote or how many followers you had or how many tech companies you worked for or how much power you wielded there or how much you vested at each. No, the biggest predictor of your happiness and fulfillment overall in life is, basically, love." According to George Vaillant, the Harvard psychiatrist who directed the study from 1972 to 2004, there are two foundational elements to this: "One is love. The other is finding a way of coping with life that does not push love away."

Love is everything, and everything is love.

—John Lennon

We can infer from the study that prioritizing our lives and making a strong network of connections is key to happiness. It is not only about having good physical health but also about having loving relationships that will ultimately make you happy. The study showed that having someone to rely on helps you relax, helps your brain stay healthier for longer, and reduces both emotional as well as physical pain.

Happiness—a symphony of harmonious balance

He who lives in harmony with himself lives in harmony with the universe.

—Marcus Aurelius

A life worth living is one that is filled with happiness most of the time. A balanced life can improve and optimize all the factors that matter to the affairs of human enterprise. Life is a journey, not a destination. We are certain that we all must die. At the end of our road, there is a clear end.

Being happy most of your life is about how you walk the road. There will be bends, curves, drops, and all sorts of tribulations along the way. How you deal with these, your outlook, the lessons you learned, how you get up, etc. — all these are what will determine your happiness level. If you learn to enjoy the journey and all its aspects, you will live a balanced life, a fulfilled life. Parameters to be optimized and mastered include mental and physical freedom, financial and material freedom, wisdom, laughter, thankfulness, generosity, virtuosity, and balance in all aspects of life. A great deal of research suggests that happiness can improve your physical health, your cardiovascular health, the immune system, inflammation levels, and blood pressure, among other things. Happiness has also been linked to improving lifespan as well as a higher quality of life.

The United States Constitution lists the pursuit of happiness as one of our most fundamental rights. Researchers have found that people from all over the world rate happiness as the most important pursuit, higher than wealth, material goods, and even physical wellbeing.

A balanced life includes a rational part of all virtues. Dan Buettner coined the term "Blue Zones" for areas of the world with the most centenarians — not only people that live longer, but who are healthier and happier. The term first appeared in his November 2005 *National Geographic* magazine story, "The Secret of a Long Life". He identified five regions a "Blue Zones": Japan (Okinawa), Italy (Sardinia), Costa Rica (Nicoya), Greece (Icaria), and California (Loma Linda). He stated that people inhabiting Blue Zones share common lifestyle characteristics that contribute to their longevity:

- Family — put ahead of other concerns.
- Less smoking.
- Semi-vegetarianism — most of the food consumed is derived from plants.
- Constant moderate physical activity — an inseparable part of life.
- Social engagement — people of all ages are socially active and integrated into their communities.
- Legumes — commonly consumed.

Buettner also lists nine lessons these people share:

1. Moderate, regular physical activity.
2. Life purpose.
3. Stress reduction.
4. Moderate caloric intake.
5. Plant-based diet.
6. Moderate alcohol intake, especially wine.
7. Engagement in spirituality or religion.
8. Engagement in family life.
9. Engagement in social life.

This study highlights some of the factors of importance in obtaining longevity and happiness. However, this list does not refer to mental and physical mastery. While the factors above are very useful tools for living a long life, they are not all-inclusive: they are missing some critical mental and physical dispositions one needs. The overarching similarities that these people all have in common are having a fit body and having a strong positive mind. A better way to measure age or longevity is to measure your number of heartbeats. Think of a car engine: a better way to assess the health of this car is to measure how many miles it has; not how old it is. If the car has been parked without being used, then it is new – low age. The human body has an average of 3.4 trillion heartbeats per lifetime. When you get your body fit and your mind healthy, your average heart rate goes down, so, in effect, you expand your lifespan. This is what we see in these centenarians, as their lifestyle is contributing to a more relaxed life and lower overall heat rates. We will look at the physical and mental parameters of happiness in a much broader and inclusive way. I will incorporate the mental-physical aspects of happiness in a more general, high-level categories. This way, one can prioritize all the factors and better understand all the components of holistic happiness. As we learn and execute all actions needed to get the best physical body we can obtain, and the clearest, healthiest mind possible, then we will reach the balance required for happiness. When breakdowns occur – the body gets ill for example – we fall out of balance and temporary happiness vanishes. If you get depressed or experience a mental breakdown of some sort, then the body breakdown follows. This is the

126

balance that one must always strive to get; only when we are in this state of balance are we in a state of happiness. This is a very delicate balance and several elements can cause the mind and body, for example, to become ill. We've already reviewed how stress affects the mind and body. We will explore the elements that affect the mental balance and study mind mastery in future chapters. The social aspects and the networks needed to be in a happy state are part of mind mastery. We have got to have healthy and productive relationships with all our networks of support; this aspect is also required to be in harmony for happiness — these are part of mental fitness.

Happiness maxim—mind and body freedom

Mind and body freedom refers to obtaining a level of wellbeing where one is healthy, fit, and free of diseases or illness. This state is obviously going to be in flux as we move in and out of fitness, but the goal is to spend most of your time on the healthy and fit side. Freedom of the body means getting your body to a state where the muscular system, the immune system, and all the other systems of the body, are working at their optimum performance — the highest level one can obtain for oneself. In a similar fashion, mind freedom is where your mind is at its optimum level of performance, free of illness and in a state of peace and clear thinking. Our daily routine should be designed to help obtain these states of freedom. Proper nutrition, exercise, an active lifestyle, social connections, life-long learning, rest, meditation, and mindfulness are all the tools that one will need to master to reach these two freedoms.

In 1943, Abraham Maslow proposed a hierarchy of needs in his paper "A Theory of Human Motivation." His hierarchy of needs has been used to study how human motivations work. It is typically shown as a pyramid with these levels: at the bottom, level I — "physiological needs"; level II — "safety needs"; level III — "belonging and love"; level IV — "social needs" or "esteem"; and level V — "self-actualization." The goal of his theory is to attain the highest level (V): self-actualization. Today, scholars prefer to think of these levels as continuously overlapping each other. A level can take priority over other levels at any point in time. By physiological needs, Maslow meant homeostasis, health, food, water, sleep, clothes, shelter, and sex. According to Maslow, these are the first step in internal motivation. If these needs are not met, the individual experiences displeasure, and they cannot move to higher levels of needs. Safety needs are the next level of needs once the physiological needs are met. Maslow's safety needs include personal security, emotional security, financial security, health and well-being, and safety needs against accidents/illness and their adverse impacts. He argues that, once a person's physiological needs have been satisfied, their safety needs take precedence and dominate the individual behavior. Safety needs are about keeping us safe from physical and or mental harm. His third level, belonging and love, is more about interpersonal relationships and involves feelings of belongingness. At this level, Maslow includes friendships, intimacy, and family. According to Maslow, humans need to feel a sense of belonging and acceptance among social groups, regardless of whether these groups are large or small. Loneliness is prevalent in modern society despite all our modern social internet connections. Many are affected by loneliness, resulting in depression and social anxiety. The fourth level, esteem, is ego or status needs. This concerns people being recognized – their sense of worth, self-esteem, and self-respect. This is the human need of being accepted and valued by others. Maslow described two versions of esteem needs: a "lower," which he refers to as the need for respect from others, and a "higher," which is the need for self-respect. The final level, self-actualization, is the realization of one's full potential. He said, "What a man can be, he must be." Maslow described this level as the desire to accomplish everything that one can, to become the most that one can be. He argues that, to get to this level, the person needs to master all previous levels. He included on this level: mate acquisition, parenting, utilizing and developing abilities, utilizing and developing talents, and pursuing goals.

To understand body freedom using Maslow's framework, one can say you accomplish body freedom once you have mastered all body-related levels of his hierarchy of needs. The need to master all these is a prerequisite to obtaining this freedom. Mind freedom similarly refers to mastering all levels of mental concerns. A level of self-actualization is presumed for one to reach these freedoms or, in other words, once you reach body and mind freedom, you will reach self-actualization. We have explored all the tools necessary to accomplish body freedom in our previous chapter on the body s a temple. The tools for mind freedom are explored further in the upcoming mind mastery chapter.

Happiness maxim—financial and material freedom

Maslow considers financial needs as a level II need on his hierarchical scale. A broader perspective for this is, instead, to consider financial freedom. Financial freedom refers to reaching a level of financial assets, money, where one does not need to work any longer to meet one basic financial need. This dollar amount will vary depending on the individual. For one person, five million dollars—investing properly to generate a 10% Return on Investing, ROI—will be enough to obtain financial freedom, while others will assess their need at hundreds of millions to reach their version of financial freedom. The actual dollar amount depends on the individuals, but we find most people grossly overestimate this number. There are several studies that show that additional financial health does not provide any corresponding increase in happiness. In contrast, consider a monk living in a convent with no financial assets to his name. For this monk, financial freedom is no monetary concerns. While I am not suggesting that we should all join a convent, I offer this example to demonstrate that financial freedom does not have to be an outrageous amount.

Once you have defined what the amount to obtain financial freedom will be for your personal situation, you develop a plan to accomplish it and focus on living in the present while simultaneously working on this goal. Financial freedom will eliminate a lot of stress associated with monetary concerns. Tony Robbins, in his book, Money Master the Game, explains seven simple steps to obtaining financial freedom. Robbins argues that one must learn to play the game. If one is going to play in the game, then one must not only know the rules of the game but master the game. He then goes on to explain that acting is super important to any action plan. Most people will not execute their plan; consequently, their plans will be just that: plans that never get done. He advises setting money aside and investing. Investing in the right portfolio is a sure way to build your financial freedom. Learn about compounding interest and how it can be used to accumulate wealth. He recommends investing like a billionaire. Billionaires invest their money in a different way than ordinary people; if one desires the returns these people get, then one must invest as they do. In the end, he said it is not about money; it is about living your best life. Money is simply a tool to help you do this. By obtaining financial freedom, this aspect of your life will be set. Remember: it is not about accumulating as much money as you can. This will just lead to a life spent in the search for wealth, and one will miss the important things of the journey. Happy people share similar traits: nurturing relationships, gratitude, helping others, being optimistic. It is not about money, material things, or beauty; it is about mindful and present living. Financial freedom can be obtained by learning all aspects of how money is made, how it is grown, and how it is invested. One will need to spend some time mastering these components. These are not exceedingly difficult and simple mathematics will allow you to put a plan together to get to your financial freedom number. Once the detailed plan is developed, one needs to execute it religiously. Financial freedom will give you peace of mind and the time to pursue all other important factors of happiness. Financial freedom is a cornerstone of your overall holistic happiness.

Material freedom is the partner of financial freedom. Material freedom refers to being free of the desires that arise from wanting more and more stuff in order to satisfy one's need to own material possessions. According to Webster-Meridian, materialism is the preoccupation with, or stress upon, material rather than intellectual or spiritual things. Our current vision of happiness is very materialistic; we need a new paradigm without materialism. In modern society, sales and marketing departments have mastered the art of creating needs where none exist. Companies, through advertisement (the average individual is exposed to over 30,000 advertisements a year), are constantly pushing products and services and making a very strong case as to why you should buy material stuff, even when the need is not there. While one can buy a functional car that satisfies all the needs this asset provides, companies spend millions to convince that you need to buy the most expensive car, even if you cannot afford it. They will provide incentives like zero percent interest rates on their financing, so that you feel that you need their specific product. The average individual does not have the intellectual capacity to see beyond their sales pitch. This applies to all material aspects of modern society, such as clothes, makeup, home products, beauty products, entertainment, and a myriad of other products. Amazon, the largest online commercial store in the world, sells about 1.7 billion products a month! Our society is one of consumerism. One obtains material freedom when one realizes these truths and learns to see beyond the attack of advertisement, simplify one's life, and use only materials that are needed for a full, balanced, and well-lived life. This does not mean a life of scarcity, but a life of moderation. This, of course, will vary depending on the individual, but material freedom is very objective, as we learn to value our relationships, wisdom, virtues, and true passions that make up a life worth living, instead of valuing the pursuit of shiny objects. This can also be thought of as the art of letting go. People cling on to material objects, as they justify themselves that this object will be of some use in the future. Letting go is hard for many; learning to live a simple existence with the essential material is a skill that we all must master. Letting go frees the mind and the soul to pursue other, higher ends. Once this level of skill is acquired, we will have achieved material freedom.

The only true wisdom is in knowing you know nothing.

—Socrates

Wisdom—application of knowledge

A life well-lived is a life with purpose and meaning. To have a purpose in life, to have meaning in one's life, one must be able to understand why what happens, happens. We have been in search of knowledge since the moment we learned to communicate complex ideas. This innate need to know is what drives us to search for meaning. Wisdom, the application of knowledge, can be obtained by being a life-long learner of scientific know-how. When we are curious, imaginative, and when we persistently chase every question and theory in a scientific way, then we have a chance to understand. The scientific method gets at the truth of the hypothesis and takes over when scientific giants have left off. We can advance our knowledge and understanding of the universe by standing on the shoulders of giants, our scientific predecessors. Knowledge leads to wisdom and wisdom leads to happiness. Sometimes people mistake knowledge for wisdom. Knowledge is more of an accumulation of facts and information, while wisdom is the synthesis of knowledge into insights that creates understanding. One can think of knowledge as a tool, and wisdom as how to use it. There is a direct correlation between wisdom and happiness: the wiser a person is, the happier he will become. It stands to reason that, if one understands the origins of most things that happen to you, around you, and to others, the better-equipped one is to deal with these things and eliminate them if they are a source of stress. Take anxiety for example. When one understands where It is coming from, then one has a chance to address it. Without this specific wisdom, one would be powerless to do anything about it. This holds for every truth that faces us during our lives. This is not to say that the unwise person is not happy, but they will have a lower level of happiness as compared to those that possess wisdom. To increase happiness, it follows, increase wisdom.

Wisdom is a learnable virtue. It can be acquired through experience, study, reflection, reading, and life-long learning. One can become wiser by learning as much as one can, about as many sciences as one can, by analyzing one's experiences, and by practicing and testing one's wisdom with others. Happiness is within reach when it is wisdom we preach.

School education is our traditional way of sharing knowledge through society. Although the acquisition is mostly formal education, it does not have to be. Informal education, through reading, experiences, and learning from others, is also enormously powerful in helping one to become knowledgeable and eventually wiser. Lack of formal education, or lack of access to it, is a form of subjugation of society, for those that do not understand, those that do not get the education, are forever slaves. However, it does not have to be that way. Applied education in all knowledge will lead to wisdom and happiness.

I cook with wine, sometimes I even add it to the food.

—W.C. Fields

Laughter—happiness panacea

The benefits of laughter are almost magical. Laughter is the ultimate stress relief and we know by now that stress is the cause of all ills. When we laugh, we produce physiological changes in our bodies which reduce our level of stress and put us in a "relaxed state". In this state, the immune system thrives. We are at our best in terms of fighting pathogens, diseases, and the healing of the body. You should laugh often, honestly, and as much as you breathe. Laugh your way to optimal health. Laughter is part of our human vocabulary. Homo sapiens understand laughter. We are born with the capacity to laugh. Laughter is unconscious — we do not decide to do it. We first start to laugh at about 3-4 months of age, long before we can speak.

It is believed that laughter evolved from the panting behavior of our ancient primate ancestors. Our laughter is often interpreted as communicating playful intent. It is a bonding function within individuals in a group. In 2005, a link between laughter and healthy function of blood vessels was reported by a researcher at the University of Maryland Medical Center. They said that laughter causes the dilation of the inner lining of blood vessels, the endothelium, and increases blood flow. Laughter has proven beneficial in several aspects of biochemistry. It has shown to reduce stress hormones such as cortisol and epinephrine. Laughter causes the brain to release endorphins that can relieve physical pain. It boosts the number of antibody-producing cells and enhances the T-cells, leading to stronger immune systems.

Researchers such as immunologist Lee S. Berk of Loma Linda University have conducted numerous clinical studies that confirm the following physiological changes when we laugh:

- The pituitary gland releases its own opiates, which suppress pain.
- The production of immune cells increases.
- The level of the hormone cortisol, which is chronically high when an individual is under long-term stress and which suppresses the immune system, is reduced dramatically.
- The level of the hormone epinephrine, which plays a role in hypertension and heart failure, decreases.
- Antibody levels in the blood and saliva rise.
- The number of natural killer cells increases, which accelerates the body's natural anticarcinogenic response.

Laughing remains a most powerful medicine. The study conducted by Dr. Berch and his colleagues found the effect that laughing has on diabetic and hypertension patients. The study had a group of twenty high-risk, diabetic patients with hypertension and hyperlipidemia. They were divided into two groups: Group C (control) and Group L (laughter). Both groups were started on standard medications for diabetes (glipizide, TZD, metformin), hypertension (ACE inhibitor or ARB), and hyperlipidemia (statins). They followed both groups for 12 months, testing their blood for the stress hormones epinephrine and norepinephrine; HDL cholesterol; inflammatory cytokines TNF-α IFN-γ and IL-6, which contribute to the acceleration of atherosclerosis and C-reactive proteins (hs-CRP), a marker of inflammation and cardiovascular disease. Group L viewed self-selected humor for 30 minutes in addition to the standard therapies described above. The patients in the laughter group (Group L) had lower epinephrine and norepinephrine levels by the second month, suggesting lower stress levels. They had increased HDL (good) cholesterol. The laughter group also had lower levels of TNF-α, IFN-γ, IL-6, and hs-CRP, indicating lower levels of inflammation. At the end of one year, the research team saw significant improvement in Group L: HDL cholesterol had risen by 26 percent in Group L (laughter), and only 3 percent in the Group C (control). Harmful C-reactive proteins decreased by 66 % in the laughter group versus 26 percent for the control group. The study suggests that the addition of an adjunct therapeutic mirthful laughter Rx (a potential modulator of positive mood state) to standard diabetes care may lower stress and inflammatory response and increase "good" cholesterol levels. The authors concluded that mirthful laughter may thus lower the risk of cardiovascular disease associated with diabetes mellitus and metabolic syndrome. Humor has scientifically been proven to improve your overall health. It is an innate response, and it is free. It is the best natural medicine I've found to aid any type of illness. Practice humor: laugh frequently and make it a major part of your daily routine. My dog teaches me laughing every day. Dog wagging is how man's best friend tells us when they are happy and content. No matter what kind of day my dog has had, no matter whether she received any food, mistreatment, or any other type of behavior, the minute I enter the door to my house I will be received with an enthusiastic dog's tail wagging. This consistent, reliable, unquestionable expression of happiness fills me with joy, and it makes me laugh. We all need to find moments, circumstances, situations, that make us laugh. Laughing is nature's gift to us, to let us know all is okay, we will be fine, if we just remember to enjoy life— if we remember to laugh.

Virtuosity—the backbone of happiness

Virtue is a state of character concerned with choice, being determined by rational principle as determined by the moderate man of practical wisdom

— Aristotle

Virtue is moral excellence. Philosophers describe a virtue as "a trait or quality that is deemed to be morally good and thus is valued as a foundation of principle and good moral being." Ever since man started living in social gatherings, there has been a concern with understanding what are the right and wrong things to do. We then started classifying certain traits as virtues and their opposites as vice. Those people that possess the virtuous traits have a high moral standard. The challenge has been to clearly define these moral standards. Who is responsible for defining these, and are they absolute or will they change over time? The creation of religion, once our languages were sophisticated enough to propagate complex ideas, helped advance the concepts of virtues. Religious people get their moral standards from their religion and also from the enforced morals of their current political and social structures. Society enforces moral standards on the individual through laws and informal punishments when morals are violated.

Benjamin Franklin had a checklist on his notebook, to check how he was living according to his virtues. The biography of Benjamin Franklin listed these as:

- **Temperance:** Eat not to Dullness. Drink not to Elevation.

- **Silence**: Speak not but what may benefit others or yourself. Avoid trifling Conversation.

- **Order**: Let all your Things have their Places. Let each Part of your Business have its Time.
- **Resolution**: Resolve to perform what you ought. Perform without fail what you resolve.

- **Frugality**: Make no Expense but to do good to others or yourself, i.e., Waste nothing.

- **Industry**: Lose no Time. Be always employed in something useful. Cut off all unnecessary Actions.

- **Sincerity**: Use no hurtful Deceit. Think innocently and justly; and, if you speak, speak accordingly.

- **Justice**: Wrong none, by doing Injuries or omitting the Benefits that are your Duty.

- **Moderation**: Avoid Extremes. Forbear resenting Injuries so much as you think they deserve.

- **Cleanliness**: Tolerate no Uncleanness in Body, Clothes or Habitation.

- **Tranquility**: Be not disturbed at Trifles, or at Accidents common or unavoidable.

- **Chastity**: Rarely use Venery but for Health or Offspring; Never to Dullness, Weakness, or the Injury of your own or another's Peace or Reputation.

- **Humility**: Imitate Jesus and Socrates.

Living a virtuous life brings enjoyment and happiness to the soul. The Dalai Lama argues that the purpose of life is to be happy. He further explains that, by practicing compassion and love, we can be on the road towards happiness. We share the planet; our "shared humanity" unites us. He mentioned that we all share an identical need for love. "Ultimately, humanity is one and this small planet is our only home, if we are to protect this home of ours, each of us needs to experience a vivid sense of universal altruism. It is only this feeling that can remove the self-centered motives that cause people to deceive and misuse one another."

One begins this journey of changes with oneself, with the person in the mirror. When one wants to create change, one needs to start with oneself. By practicing virtuosity in all its aspects, by starting with oneself, one starts making little ripples in the water; when enough ripples are made, a tsunami is created — a brand new joyful world. This is the Efenian's way. An Efenian is a virtuous individual.

Food is Thy Medicine

Let food be thy medicine, and let medicine be thy food

— Hippocrates

H ippocrates, one of the greatest physicians of antiquity (460-370 BC), is the most influential figure in the history of medicine and referred to as the father of western medicines. He was born on the island of Kos, Greece. Not a lot is known about his life. According to Aristotle's testimony, he was known as "The Great Hippocrates." He was usually portrayed as a kind, dignified, old country doctor. He was of great intellect and generally regarded as very wise. Fielding Garrison, a medical historian, stated, "He is, above all, the exemplar of that flexible, critical, well-poised attitude of mind, ever on the lookout for sources of error, which is the very essence of the scientific spirit."

Hippocrates lived during Greece's classical period. It has been arduous to separate the facts from the fiction when it comes to his life, as he was so highly revered that sometimes the stories morphed into tales. During his lifetime, he was admired as a physician and as a great teacher. Plato referred to him in two of his dialogs, *Protagoras* and *Phaedrus*. Plato implied that Hippocrates was a great physician with a philosophical approach to medicine. Meno, a pupil of Aristotle, stated that Hippocrates believed the undigested residues were produced by an unsuitable diet and that these residues excreted vapors which passed to the body and produced diseases. Aristotle called him "the Great Physician", but he further added small in politics. Hippocrates is known to have traveled extensively in Greece and Asia Minor practicing his art of medicine and teaching students. His reputation and myth took off one hundred years after his death. The Museum of Alexandria in Egypt collected his works in celebration of the past greatness of Greece. His great body of medical works was assembled as a group called the works of Hippocrates — *Corpus hippocraticum.* All the virtues of classical medical works were eventually attributed to him.

There is no doubt that Hippocrates was a great physician with tremendous influence on the development of this field, one who also practiced optimum physician ethics and ideals. There are over 60 medical writings that have survived which are attributed to him. He is frequently associated with the ideal physician. Hippocrates understood the power of food and recommended its use to cure diseases. He often used lifestyle modifications such as diet and exercise to treat diseases such as diabetes. The Hippocratic Oath, credited to him, put demands on doctors to uphold the profession to the highest standards of the times. For example: "I will use those dietary regimens which will benefit my patients . . . and I will do no harm or injustice to them." The original oath has been modified somewhat, but contrary to popular belief, most modern doctors never take this oath. He is also attributed with the saying, "Let food be thy medicine and medicine be thy food." This two-thousand-year-old aphorism still rings true today. The virtues of his writing are many and all revolved around eschewing technical jargon and, instead, focusing on the earnest desire to help the patient.

FOOD IS THY MEDCINE

The Hippocratic Corpus is a collection of some 60 works. Amongst them is *On Airs, Waters, Places* in which, instead of using traditional claims to the divine origin, he focused on the environmental causes. It proposed that considerations such as weather, water drinking, and sites along the paths of favorable winds can help a physician ascertain the general health of citizens. Several of his work advanced the revolutionary idea that, by observing enough cases, a physician can predict the course of a disease. On *Regiment and Regimen in Acute Diseases*, he conceived the idea of preventive medicine. He not only stressed diet but also how the patient's general way of living influences their health and convalescence. *Sacred Disease, a treatise on epilepsy* reveals the rudimentary knowledge, and lack thereof, of anatomy of the times. It was believed at that time that epilepsy was caused by insufficient air, which was thought to be carried by the veins to the brain and limbs. Wholesome foods heal and repair the body. Real and wholesome foods not only provide the nutrients that the body and microbiome need to grow and reproduce, but also provide a host of many vital chemicals the body needs to function optimally. The healing power of nutrition is a balanced combination of multiple supporting roles that synergistically work together. 'Let food be thy medicine' refers to maintaining this beautiful balance. By consuming all types of organic foods that the body needs, one supports the structure and function of the brain and the physical body. The brain and the guts control our moods and emotions. Foods we eat feed the brain and the body so, in turn, our foods determine our physical and mental state. You are what you eat.

CHAPTER 10: A COCKTAIL OF ROSES

FOOD — NATURE'S MEDICINE

Do not eat anything your great-great-grandmother wouldn't recognize as food"

— Michael Pollan

L ightning violently and loudly struck a dry branch on the open savanna and started an out of control fire that stunned our early ancestor, as this was their first encounter with the lively flame. To the early humans, the heat and destructive power of fire demanded god-like status. It is only after Homo erectus, during the early Stone Age, that our descendants started to understand the essence of fire. Early humans started mastering fire and using it for cooking and softening their source of proteins — the tough meat of other early animals. The earliest evidence of controlled fire associated with humans comes from Oldowan hominin sites in the Lake Turkana region of Kenya. The Australopithecine site of Chesowanja, in central Kenya, 1.4 million years old, also showed evidence of controlled fire by humans. Archeologists have concluded, based on the available evidence, that habitual use of fire was not part of the human behavior until about 300,000 to 400,000 years ago. They believe that the earlier sites of controlled fire are representative of the opportunistic use of natural fires. Terrence Twomey published a comprehensive discussion of the evidence of early fire. He believes that there is no direct evidence for domestic fires between 400,000 and 700,000 years ago, but he believes that other, indirect evidence supports the notion of the controlled use of fire. Gowlett and R. Wrangham argue that another piece of indirect evidence for the early use of fire is that our ancestors Homo erectus evolved smaller mouths, teeth, and digestive systems, in striking contrast to earlier hominids. The benefits of having a smaller gut could not be realized until high-quality foods were available. Fire for cooking softens the food and makes it easier to digest. This change to food, cooking, could have led to those phenotypical changes.

Fire, fuel of growth — progenitor of man's food

Fire ignited a revolution for early humans in the cooking of food and would eventually change the nature of humanity. The discovery of fire, and the taming of it, is one of the earliest game-changers created by man. Fire allowed our early ancestors to cook food, thus making available a brand-new range of easy to digest meats and plants which would end up evolving our early brain into the highly tuned brain of modern humans.

For animals in the wild, food is just food; for Homo sapiens food is much more. It is family, socializing, economy, environment, culture – it is life. Food is generally defined as any nutritious substance that people or animals eat or drink in order to maintain life and growth. The acquisition, preparation, and consumption of food are intimately connected with what it is like to be human. This process creates bonds that last a lifetime. Our relationship with food is a long one; it dates to the very first-time humans became self-aware.

Cooking is at once child's play and adult joy.

And cooking done with care is an act of love.

— Craig Claiborne

Cooking is not only the addition of heat from the fire but also includes the chopping and grinding of the food. Cooking breaks down collagen, the connective tissue in meat, and softens the cell walls of plants to release the sources of nutritious starch and fats. As the quality of food and ease of digestion increased, the brain kept evolving. The calories to fuel bigger brains of successive species of hominids came at the expense of the energy-intensive tissue in the gut, which was shrinking at the same time. One can see that the barrel-shape trunk of the apes morphed into the comparatively narrow-wasted Homo sapiens. Cooking provided additional time — by eliminating the additional chewing needed — for other activities that promote the growth of the brain. The great apes spend four to seven hours a day just chewing. Fire transformed the human evolution of our early ancestors and gave us the brain sizes we currently possess. The use of fire made us more human.

Cooking evolved throughout human history to the form of mass feeding we presently practice. From the early form of cooking around a fire to the later modern kitchen, cooking has forged vital bonds for the highly sociable Homo sapiens. The social aspects of the cooking process are as important as the nutritional ones. By sharing cooking and the eating of foods, families communicate their values, fears, competition strategies, survival, and reproduction concerns. The cooking tradition in modern cities is vanishing as quickly as conveniences are appearing. When one cooks with families and friends, camaraderie is strengthened — the body and the soul rejoice as they about to receive the nourishment that comes from a place of knowledge of all ingredients and process, from a place where there is enough love, to create food.

Gathering food at light speed

Early humans secured food by hunting and gathering, and eventually, agriculture came onto the scene. This prehistoric selection of meats and plants gave modern humans their mainly omnivorous diet. Throughout history, humans have significantly increased their cuisines to include a great variety of ingredients: herbs, spices, and all sorts of plants and meats. During the Middle Ages, which began in Europe after the fall of the Roman Empire and lasted for almost a thousand years, most of the food was homegrown. In this time, the food was controlled by the seasons, the environment, and the Church. Poor families ate a diet of vegetables in the form of stew, soup, or pottage. They were not allowed to hunt deer, boar, or rabbits as could members of the noble class. Species were a privilege of the upper classes. The staple items of the poor included rye or barley bread, stews, local dairy products, cheaper meats like beef, pork or lamb, some fish, and homegrown herbs, if available. Grains like bread, beer, oats, and root vegetables were grown for stews, and animals were raised for both meat and other products like wool, leather, etc. Fruits, nuts, and honey from local trees were also part of the diet of the times, when available. Food was cooked over an open fire or pit. Their ovens were made from some form of clay. Poor families during these times were unable to obtain nutritious or varied food. This period was filled with wars, poverty, isolation, and struggles for survival. For the upper class and noble families, the struggles were not as severe.

During what is called the long-18th century (1685-1815), Europe moved out of the Dark Ages and into the age of the Enlightenment. Some consider the publication of Isaac Newton's Principia Mathematica (1687) as the first major work of this era. Grain and livestock had been the most important agricultural products in France and England. After 1700, new and innovative farming techniques started to increase yield and look into new products such as hops, oilseed rape, artificial grasses, vegetables, fruit, day foods, commercial poultry, rabbits and freshwater fish. Sugar began to be produced in Caribbean sugar plantations, worked by African slaves, as an upper-class luxury product. By 1800, sugar was a staple of working-class diets. During the American colonial era (1600 to 1700), the diets of early settlers came from small farms which were known as the "breadbasket colonies" because they grew so many crops, such as wheat, barley, oats, rye, and corn. They farmed pumpkins, beans, and squash. The colonies also had access to fish and seafood, like tuna, cod, trout, clams, salmon, oysters, and mussels. They hunted game birds and other small prey. The food of this time consisted of three meals a day. Breakfast would be bread or cornmeal with milk and or tea. Dinner, usually in the middle of the day, would include meats, vegetables, and dessert. Super, during the evening, would be a smaller meal, like bread and cheeses, pudding, or leftovers from the noon meal. Without refrigeration, the food would be preserved using salt, pickling, drying, smoking, and making preserves such as marmalades, jams, and syrups. Some herbs of the time were basil, lovage, mint, parsley, sage, and dill. They also enjoyed coffee, tea, and chocolate drinks. Food did not change much during the 18th century. Despite improvements in farming, food for the common man remained plain and monotonous. For many of them, meat was a luxury. The poor person's diet was mostly bread and potatoes.

The food variety and quantity improved as the 19th century rolled around. Meat was still a luxury, and the working class was eating mostly plain food such as bread, butter, potatoes, and bacon. However, new technologies, like the railways, steamboats, and refrigeration, changed food availability by leaps and bounds. These technologies made possible the importation of cheap meat from Australia and Argentina. Sugar consumption increased greatly. By the end of the 19th century, most people were eating better. The first fish and chip shops in Britain opened in the 1860s. They soon became very common in British towns and cities. The immigrant in the early United States brought with them their food cooking styles and cultures. Housewives were able to buy ready-made food from street peddlers, from pushcarts, and from small shops operating from private homes. This made possible new items such as pizza, spaghetti with meatballs, bagels, hoagies, pretzels, and perogies, and thus established the onset of fast food in America. By the end of this century, canned food became widely available. Several new inventions accelerated the fast food industry: William Lyman invented the rotary can opener in 1870, Hippolyte Mege-Mouries invented margarine—a cheap substitute for butter — milk chocolate was invented in 1875, and the first recipe for potato crisps — potato chips — was published in 1817. The first electric oven hit the United States market in 1891.

Food in the 20th century fluctuated wildly as humanity became involved in two world wars. During wartime, starvation of civilian population was sometimes used as a weapon. After the end of World War II, new food products became more readily available to the masses, and with it came a proliferation of branded foods and advertisements. Now, instead of spending hours in the kitchen, the housewife could purchase instant foods in jars, or ready-mixed powders. The well-to-do had ice boxes — thus changing the storage of food and the amount of food they need to buy at a time — and the era of food convenience started. This century saw the development of what some called the Third Agricultural Revolution — The Green Revolution. Several initiatives launched in the 1950s and 1960s lead to increased agricultural worldwide production, particularly in the developing world. The initiatives included high-yielding varieties of cereals, especially dwarf wheat and rice, associated with chemical fertilizers and agro-chemicals, controlled irrigation, cultivation mechanization — all these together were to supersede traditional agricultural techniques.

In 1912, Joseph Horn and Frank Hardart opened an automat in New York. It would become a sensation, and most historians have pinned it as the start of a food revolution in America — the fast-food industry. They had opened their first automat in Philadelphia (1902), but the New York one would be their most successful one. Several other automats were opened around the country to feed the high demand for that type of service. Automats also made popular the notion of "take-out" food, with the slogan "Less work for mother." The fast-food industry is thought of as a specific type of restaurant that serves food in a relatively fast time with minimal table service. The automat was a cafeteria-style food prepared behind small glass windows and with coin-operated slots. It was followed by a series of industrial improvements and innovations all destined to increase the speed of food delivery while providing cheap and somewhat reasonable quality food. The food was from a limited menu, cooked in bulk, kept hot, finished and packaged to order. The meaning of food evolved through the centuries and metamorphosed on par with the proliferation of technology, population growth, and food demands. Some historians argued that White Castle was the first fast-food restaurant, starting in Wichita, Kansas in 1916, selling hamburgers for five cents. William Ingram and Walter Anderson created the first fast-food supply chain which provided meat, buns, paper goods, and other supplies for their stores. The McDonald's 'Speedee Service System,' Ray Kroc's McDonald's outlets, and Hamburger University were all built on White Castle practices, systems, and principles.

The birth of the fast-food industry is considered one of the largest and most radical changes in the food industry, and its negative impact on the overall health of the country has been mammoth. Fast-food is not only the kind that comes out of the fast-food restaurants, but it includes chips, sodas, cookies, candy, breakfast cereals, French fries, burgers, pizza, white flour baked goods, and all other high-calorie, nutrient-poor foods that people eat multiple times during the day. These foods do not need to be prepared, can be accessed quickly and easily, come in a bag or box ready to go into your mouth, and are very quickly absorbed into the bloodstream. They usually contain several added artificial chemicals and synthetic ingredients to prolong their shelf life and enhance flavors. Typical ingredients include artificial sweeteners, salt, coloring agents, corn syrup, sugar, and other potentially disease-causing chemicals. Since the inception of the fast-food industry, the health of Americans has progressively decreased, resulting in epidemic levels of chronic maladies. 71 percent of Americans are overweight or obese, as compared to just 66 percent five years ago. The consumption of processed food and fast-food is estimated to kill more people prematurely than cigarette smoking. There is a direct correlation between the amount of fast-food, processed food, sugars, and the destruction of brain cells, which consequently leads to diminishing brain capacity, lowered intelligence. Multiple studies have shown that higher amounts of animal product consumption may lead to premature aging, increased risk of chronic disease, higher all-cause mortality. Animal products served at fast-food restaurants are decreasing the overall health of the population, creating dangerous carcinogens from being fried at high temperatures. The World Health

Association has classified processed meats — hot dogs, sausage, bacon, and lunch meats — as class-1 carcinogens. Refined carbohydrates are not only related to overweight, diabetes, and heart disease but they also contribute to dementia, mental illness, and cancer. Refined carbohydrates include rice, sugar, maple syrup, and agave nectar, just to name a few.

The fast-food industry has also led to an increase in the amount of food consumed by the average American. The sugar content, coupled with the seemingly low price of the so-called food, has led people to over-consume calories. Research has shown that excess calorie consumption leads to a shortened lifespan, whereas consuming moderate to low calories slows down the aging process and protects the body and the brain. Americans consume more calories than any other country, and most of these calories are nutrient-poor and calorie-dense foods. Fast-foods are no doubt tastier than ever, convenient and quick to get, and the price of buying them is as cheap as its nutritional quality; however, fast-foods are slowly and steadily single-handedly destroying the health of entire civilizations and humanity's health has suffered because of it.

Today, the food industry has become industrialized and all the aspects of socialization related to food have been diminishing as fast as the quality of the food itself. While industrialization paved the way to feed billions of people, it came at a high cost: human health. Profit became more important than nutrition, and corporations acquired a more dominant position in the food we ultimately consume. An article in *Business Insider Magazine* argues that only ten companies control almost every large food and beverage brand in the world! These companies are Nestlé, PepsiCo, Coca-Cola, Unilever, Danone, General Mills, Kellogg's, Mars, Associated British Foods, and Mondelez. These companies employ thousands and make billions of dollars in revenue every year. When such a small number of companies own an entire market segment, the opportunity for conflict of interest between the consumer and them is almost assured.

Fat and sugar, friend or foe?

1910 was not a significant year of the 20th-century – except that it would birth one of the most significant figures in the fat-sugar debate – Dr. John Yudkin. Yudkin was raised in the East End of London in an Orthodox Jewish family that fled the Russian pogroms of 1905. The years between Queen Victoria's death (1901) and the onset of the First World war (1914) were years of growth and, in general, good prosperity. However, wealth inequality between the Victorians and the poor, typical of this period, was significant. By 1900, London had a population of five million – one out of five Britons lived in London – but the number had ballooned to seven million by 1911. The tenth decade in London was characterized by the burgeoning Women's Suffrage movement. Led by Emmeline Pankhurst and the Women's Social and Political Union, many protests and demonstrations took place in the city, reaching the peak when the movement militarized in 1914. Hyde Park hosted two major suffragette rallies, with over 250,000 attendees. Young John Yudkin had only his mother, as his father died when he was just six years old. His mother, ridden with poverty, had to raise John and his brothers Michael, Jonathan, and Jeremy, all by herself. John managed to get a scholarship to Hackney Downs School. The school had 600 boys by the early 1970s. Its notable alumni included Nobel prize-winning playwright Harold Pinter, tycoon John Bloom, and playwright Steven Berkoff. John continued his study by securing another scholarship to Chelsea Polytechnic and, finally, to Christ's College, Cambridge, where he studied physiology and biochemistry. After earning his BS in Science, John briefly considered becoming a teacher – but decided instead to pursue a scholarship to the University of Cambridge. John's exceptional intelligence would impress the eminent bacteriologist of the time, Marjorie Stephenson, so that she offered to fund him out of her pocket while he studied with her for his Ph.D. Marjorie was a British biochemist who did pioneer research in bacterial metabolism. She was one of the first two women elected a Fellow of the Royal Society. Yudkin came to international attention while working in her research lab. His Ph.D. thesis was on "adaptive enzymes". His account of these processes inspired the research of Jacques Monod, who went to work out the detailed mechanism for the induction of enzymes in bacteria and was awarded the Nobel Prize for his work. During this time, Yudkin started to explore his interest in nutrition, a passion that he nurtured throughout his entire career.

⁂

1n 1933, Yudkin married the love of his life, Milly Himmelweit, only a few weeks after meeting her. Milly left Berlin to escape the worsening political environment of what was becoming Nazi Germany. She became his constant support and adviser. Their marriage would last for over 60 years, until her death in March 1995 — John would never be the same after Milly departed.

In 1934, while working in Ph.D. research, Yudkin commenced medical studies and started teaching physiology and biochemistry to medical students. He began clinical studies at The London Hospital, in 1935, while teaching in Cambridge during the weekends. After completing his medical studies, he was appointed Director of Medical Studies at Christ's College. During this same year, he started research at the Dunn Nutritional Laboratory, in Cambridge, working on the effects of dietary vitamins. His studies of the nutritional status of school children in Cambridge showed that supplementation of the diet with vitamins had little effect on their general health. The studies also showed that children from a poorer area of Cambridge were shorter and lighter, and had lower hemoglobin levels and a weaker grip, than those from a wealthier area. John realized that nutrition was not only a biological science but that it had especially important socio-political implications.

As World War II rolled in, Yudkin served in the Royal Army Medical Corps and was posted to Sierra Leone. During his post — he studied a skin disease that was prevalent among local African soldier — she discovered the disease was not an infection, as suspected, but instead, a riboflavin deficiency. He found that the diet which the army created was adequate for all nutrients, including riboflavin, which came primarily from millet. However, it turns out that millet was disliked by Sierra Leone soldier, who would not consume it even at the risk of starving. Yudkin started then to understand the connection between social customs and the choice of food people consume. The correlation between the food people eat and body health was becoming apparent. After World War II ended, Yudkin returned to academia. He was elected to the Chair of Physiology at Queen Elizabeth College in London. He would go to form a BSc degree in nutrition – the first degree in nutrition in any European university.

The country in 1950 was abandoning the food rationing policies of wartimes. Consequently, people started to metamorphize into obese beings due to the apparent food abundance. The manufacturing food industry expanded greatly during this time; refined sugar became a crucial ingredient in a very wide range of products, and in creating an image of an abundance ready-made convenience foods. Yet, as sugar was being added to all these products, rates of diabetes, obesity, and heart diseases were quietly escalating. Slimming diets were proliferating like weeds. Yudkin argued that, for most patients, weight could be controlled by restricting dietary carbohydrates. His interest in sugar started during these observations and was propelled by the increase of incidence of coronary thrombosis. This increase was attributed at the time to the amount of fat in the diet. Yudkin analyzed diets and coronary mortality rates in the United Kingdom between 1928 and 1954. Consequently, he published a paper stating that no evidence for the view that total fat, or animal fat, or hydrogenated fat, was the direct cause of coronary thrombosis; in fact, he states, the closest relationship between coronary deaths and any single dietary factor was with "sugar." A secondary paper by Yudkin suggested that changes in lifestyle – reduced exercise, another diet factor other than fat – during the past decades were contributing to the increased incidence of coronary deaths.

Sugar, which provides calories but not nutrients, was a clear culprit for the obesity trend and the trends of coronary disease. Sugar consumption dramatically increased during these periods. Yudkin started to conclude that excessive sugar in the diet was not only causing obesity but was also responsible for coronary heart diseases. He found that the wealthier the country, the higher the sugar consumption in the form of all additional process products and additives. In 1964, he wrote, "In the wealthier countries, there is evidence that sugar and sugar-containing foods contribute to several diseases, including obesity, dental caries, diabetes mellitus and myocardial infarction (heart attack)." The medical belief of this time was that sugar and starch both metabolized in the same way. Thus, they did not expect any difference in the effects of these two.

However, Yudkin and the team conducted experiments on animals and on human volunteers and showed that there were major differences between the two carbohydrates in their metabolic effects. As far back as 1967, Yudkin's work was demonstrating that excessive consumption of sugar may result in a disturbance in the secretion of insulin and that this, in turn, might contribute to atherosclerosis and diabetes.

In 1972, Yudkin published his famous book, *Pure, White, and Deadly*. In it, he summarizes the evidence that the consumption of sugar was leading to an increased incidence of coronary thrombosis, that it correlated with dental caries, obesity, diabetes, liver disease, and possibly with gout, dyspepsia, and some cancers. He wrote, "I hope that when you have read this book, I shall have convinced you that sugar is really dangerous." As expected, this was not well received by the sugar industry and its associated processed food manufacturers. They started a campaign to destroy Yudkin's reputation and to discredit his work. In 1955, US President Dwight Eisenhower suffered a heart attack. Instead of remaining quiet about the incident, Eisenhower insisted on sharing with the public his unfortunate event. The following day, his chief physician, Dr. Paul Dudley White, gave a press conference detailing to the American public how to prevent heart attacks. In his speech, Dr. Dudley instructed Americans that, in order to avoid heart attacks, they should stop smoking and cut down on fat and cholesterol. He cited the research of the American physiologist, Ancel Benjamin Keys.

Ancel Keys was born in Colorado Springs in 1904. Two years later, his father, Benjamin Pious Keys, and mother, Carolyn Emma Chaney, moved to San Francisco, before the great 1906 San Francisco earthquake; shortly after that, they relocated to Berkeley, where Keys would grow up and go to school. Ancel Keys was a very smart boy; as a matter of fact, he was considered to be a gifted youngster. He would do odd jobs during his high school years and eventually end up going to the University of

California at Berkeley in 1922. At UC Berkeley, Keys studied chemistry, but was unhappy and decided to take some time off; he took a job as an oiler aboard the S.S. President Wilson. He got a chance to travel abroad on this assignment to China. Eventually, he would return to Berkeley and finished his studies and graduate in B.A. in economics and political science and an M.S. in zoology. After a short time away in which he took a job as a management trainee at Woolworth's, he returned to UC Berkeley to get his Ph.D. in oceanography and biology. He was awarded a National Research Council fellowship that took him to Copenhagen, Denmark, where he worked in zoology for a couple of years. Once his fellowship ended, he took some time to teach at Harvard University, after which he went to Cambridge where he earned a second Ph.D. in physiology in 1936.

〜

In 1956, Keys launched his famous *The Seven Countries Study*, with a yearly grant of $200,000 USD from the US Public Health Service. The study was an epidemiological longitudinal one, examining the relationship between lifestyle, diet, coronary heart diseases, and stroke in different populations from different regions of the world. It focused attention on the root cause of coronary heart disease and stroke. The study was first published in 1978 and then followed up on its subjects every five years thereafter. Based on his studies, Keys claimed that fat was to blame for the rise in heart diseases, and only a diet low in fat would lower cholesterol and reverse the current trend prevalent now across the Western Worlds. The Seven Countries Study suggested that the risk and rate of heart attack and stroke correlated directly and independently to the level of total serum cholesterol in the seven sample countries. Keys was highly charismatic and combative. A colleague described him as "direct to the point of bluntness, critical to the point of skewering;" others were not as charitable.

Keys was able to convince the President of the United States and the public at large that fatty foods were unhealthy. Doctors soon joined the bandwagon, and this concept became ingrained in the general medical dogma. Many scientists were skeptical of Keys' conclusion, amongst them, John Yudkin. Yudkin had done several studies and had observed that sugar, not fat, was the culprit. Keys was very aware of Yudkin's hypothesis. He called Yudkin's hypothesis of sugar "a mountain of nonsense" and accused Yudkin of issuing "propaganda" for the meat and dairy industries. Yudkin never responded in a manner to this accusation, as he was mild-mannered and unskilled in the art of political rhetoric. The British Sugar Bureau diminished Yudkin's hypothesis, as well, and called it "emotional assertions." The World Sugar Research Organization called his book "science fiction." Keys continued to accumulate political favors, and, throughout the decades of the sixties, he secured a place for himself and his allies on the boards of the most influential bodies in American healthcare, including the American Heart Association and the National Institute of Health. Keys' hypothesis—the fat hypothesis— became the norm in America's medical system and with the public at large. It turned out; however, the whole Seven Country Study was flawed and statistically insignificant. There was no objective basis for the countries selected for the study, and Keys literally handpicked only those countries that favored his data. The study left out countries like France and Germany, which Keys knew had relatively low rates of heart disease, despite living on a diet rich in saturated fats. In spite of questionable statistical evidence, the study became the gospel by which the government dictated its policies. Dietary guidelines, headed by Senator George McGovern, were written under the premise of the fat hypothesis.

Efforts of the sugar industry to discredit Yudkin were largely successful. His reputation was destroyed. He found himself uninvited to nutrition conferences, and journals refused his papers. He was talked about by fellow scientists as an eccentric and loner. Sheldon Reiser, one of the few researchers still working on the refined carbohydrates said that, "John was so discredited He was ridiculed in a way. And anybody else who said something bad about sugar, they would say, he's just like John." By the time of Yudkin's death in 1995, his warning was no longer being taken seriously.

Forty years later, John would be vindicated by science. Robert Lustig, a pediatric endocrinologist at the University of California, in a 90-minute talk he gave in 2009, entitled *Sugar: The Bitter Truth,* argues that fructose, a sugar, is a "poison" culpable of America's obesity epidemic. Upon reading John Yudkin's book he commented, "Holy crap, this guy got there 35 years before me," referring to John's hypothesis on sugar. John has finally been recognized for the genius he was and Keys for the politician he embodied.

Processed sugars are the real cause of most chronic diseases. The sugar industry, in conjunction with the beverage and food industry, has been hiding the truth from the general public for decades. One can take a page from the cigarette industry which denied the cancerous nature of cigarettes for decades. Similarly, the sugar industry has denied the poisonous effect of excessive processed sugar consumption. They have sung the tune that a calorie is a calorie. The argument implied is that the source of calories is of no importance. The "zero-calorie" was birthed from this assumption. The conundrum with this hypothesis is that it is absolutely wrong. One calorie of sugar is not the same as a calorie, let us say, of protein. The body metabolizes both of these nutrients in a completely different fashion. Unfortunately, the marketing arm of the sugar industry is highly proficient at communication and selling their views. A popular advertisement for the famous brand Coca Cola describes opening a can of cola as "Open Happiness." The general public relates the drinking of this sugary beverage to being happy: clearly deceitful advertising, as sugar is toxic to the body in a relatively small amount. One should look to eliminate all processed sugar from one's diet and, instead, replace it with natural sugar from eating whole foods like fruits and vegetables.

Fats are essential to creating a naturally fit body: fats do not make you fat, sugars do. Fats from butter, lards, coconut oil, olive oils, and nuts are all essential for the optimum functioning body, and one should get a regular dosage of all these fats. On the other hand, one should avoid all industrially processed fats like margarine, hydrogenated and partially hydrogenated oil—soy, canola, corn, cottonseed, etc. Visceral fat, belly fat, is very detrimental to one's health. The body is very good at storing fat in times of plenty. Insulin is the hormone in charge of this mechanism. When insulin is produced, glucose is moved from the blood to the various cells in the body. Insulin is produced whenever we have glucose in our body. This hormone is sometimes referred to as the growth hormone, since it promotes the absorption of the sugar into the cell, producing the visceral fat that we are most familiar with. This fat around the midsection is the hardest to get rid of as it is the last source that the body goes to. The body first uses all available calories, and only when there is no energy anywhere else does it reach out for the reserves of fat. Fatty liver is a condition caused by excessive fat in the liver tissue. Fasting, exercising, and proper nutrition are the key tools needed to remove visceral fats. Only these work in a long term, sustainable manner.

Eschew medicinal drugs—nature's food suffices

There is substantial scientific evidence that diet plays an important role in the development and treatment of numerous chronic maladies. One such paper was published in the *European Journal of Clinical Nutrition* on the health outcomes of the Mediterranean diet. The goal of this study was to investigate the association between adherence to the Mediterranean diet and 37 different health outcomes. The study included thirteen meta-analyses of observational studies and randomized clinical trials (RCTs). Researchers found that greater adherence to the Mediterranean diet is associated with a reduced risk of major chronic diseases. They found a reduced risk of overall mortality, cardiovascular diseases, coronary heart disease, myocardial infarction, overall cancer incidence, neurodegenerative diseases, and diabetes. Researchers found that the prevalence of overweight and obesity was inversely associated with this diet. For site-specific cancers, as well as for inflammatory and metabolic parameters, they found the evidence to be suggestive or weak. The Mediterranean diet is generally characterized by high consumption of plant foods—fruits, vegetables, legumes, nuts and seeds, and wholegrain cereals. The produces used are preferably locally sourced. Daily desserts are mainly fruits. Olive oil is the primary source of lipids. Consumption of dairy products—mostly cheeses and yogurt—is moderate. Fish, poultry, and eggs are consumed in low to moderate amounts. Red meat is consumed in small amounts, and low frequency, and a moderate intake of wine is included during meals. This diet is low in saturated and trans fats, with optimal nutritional quality due to the presence of healthy fats from olive oil, nuts, fish, as well as complex carbohydrates, micronutrients, antioxidants, and, furthermore, it is abundant in fiber from varied plant-based composition with enough protein from both plant and animal origin. The Mediterranean diet has not only been held as a health model but is also praised as a cultural model. It is highly palatable and affordable. It results in lower environmental footprints due to its greater emphasis on plant-based foods rather than animal-based ones.

Foods provide all the nutrients that the body and the mind need to survive, thrive, and ultimately heal. Unfortunately, medications have become the answer to all problems—a panacea to any maladies. Although there is no doubt that some medicines can save lives, especially in cases of chronic or emergency situations, they are currently being used indiscriminately and with the purpose of alleviating symptoms. Medications do not address the root cause of maladies. They rarely prevent diseases. People are taking more medication than at any other time in our history, yet the number of sick people is not decreasing. Fifty percent of Americans have a least one chronic disease and the number is growing. Medications are a ridiculously small part of the solution. A better solution is a preventive approach where one makes the body strong by proper nutrition and exercise, and by reducing the prevailing damaging level of current stress. Natural wholesome food should become the focus: medicines should be rarely used—only in a case where a natural holistic solution is not possible. A few research institutions are starting to realize the importance that food plays in the proper function of the body and they are deciphering the thousands and thousands of chemicals contained in the food that affect our body and mind in ways we have yet to understand. The only supplement one needs is varied and diverse natural foods.

It has been scientifically proven that you can heal yourself. In *Mind over Medicine*, Dr. Lissa Rankin details the proven ways in which one can heal oneself from just about any condition, with proper nutrition, rest, meditation, and overall increasing your immune system strength. She reviews the placebo effects and the strength of positive thinking in addressing all types of ills. She affirms that our minds have the power to heal us. If we believe that we can be healed, chances are that we will. On the psychological effects, she states that happiness is preventive medicine, while loneliness poisons the body. Studies have shown that happier people live longer than unhappy ones. In one of her studies, she described the story of nurses going through cancer therapies, and the conclusion of the study showed that nurses who went through cancer alone were found to be four times more likely to die from their disease than those with ten or more friends supporting their journey. Through her research, she discovered that patients who are given placebos do not just feel better — they can actually become clinically better. Dr. Rankin's great insight is the recognition that the body has an innate ability to self-repair and that we can control this self-healing mechanism with the power of the mind.

Only sick people need medicine: a healthy individual has no need for artificial medicines. Drugs are designed to alleviate some symptoms but, in general, they do not cure the illness itself. This applies to over-the-counter (OTC) medicines as well, as they also only provide temporary relief for symptoms but do not address the real cause of the body breakdown. If the medicine cured the illness, there would be no need to continue taking it. Unfortunately, the highest percentage of our current medical system is managing symptoms; what is needed instead is health promotion. A healthy individual considers food as its source of medicine to prevent and cure most of the prevailing maladies. Superfoods like garlic, berries, tomatoes, and so forth, all contain bioactive chemicals whose healing mechanisms we have yet to understand. But the actual benefits have been scientifically quantified. When we refer to food as your medicine, this is what we mean: making sure one is including a varied source of nutrition that contains all the needed nutrients to keep the body free of illness and in a general healthy fit state. The color of the food is a good indicator of the nutrient profile of the food. By ensuring a colorful plate, we are covering all the basics and giving ourselves the best chance to get all nutrients needed. Scientists have found, for example, that vitamin B may protect against harmful epigenetic effects of pollution and may be able to combat the harmful effects that particular matter has on the body. Air pollution alters the methyl tags on DNA and increases one's risk of neurodegenerative diseases.

Plant-based nutrition—the best option

A simple rule to help with the selection of nutrition is *"If a man makes it do not eat it."* When we introduce artificial chemicals with the purpose of extending the shelf life of the product, altering the taste profile, or when we isolate only specific chemicals (i.e., supplements), we are missing hundreds of other naturally occurring chemicals that are available to the product in its natural form. Consider synthetic apple juice as a typically processed product. Apples contain a wide variety of phytochemicals, many of which have been found to have strong antioxidants and anticancer activity. Apples have been found to decrease the risk of cancer, cardiovascular diseases, and asthma, as well as to decrease lipid oxidation, and to lower cholesterol. When we consume the apple whole, including its peel, we get access to all the bioactive ingredients. However, if we opt for the processed alternative, the juice, then we are only getting a fraction of the available phytochemicals. Processing of apples has been found to affect phytochemical content. Synthetic foods were created with the idea of feeding a large number of people, which in principle is good and noble; however, profit targets and misguided direction has made the maximization of profit the primary goal of corporations. This has resulted in the overwhelming number of processed products we see in our modern supermarkets – over one hundred thousand products. Parameters like shell life, ease of distribution, low cost, and easily reproducible commodities became the key levers of the food industry. The conversation of feeding masses with the optimal nutritional food was left in the background and the profit optimization took center stage. As a result, the end product – highly processed food – became highly profitable, achieving the goals of a few, and the nutrition value of this food was relegated to second class importance. This is why, if man makes it, we do not eat it. Look for whole-food: foods that are nutrient-rich, varied, of many different colors, and locally produced. Synthetic chemicals were the backbones of the industrial revolution. These products were manufactured to make our life easier, to keep us safe from microbes, and keep us in better health. Unfortunately, none of those claims was ever fulfilled. The trend of chronic diseases keeps increasing in direct proportion to these life-simplifying, synthetic products.

Prepare food in its most natural form for maximum nutritional value: Processed food is loaded with preservatives; food additives, to enhance flavor and promote consumption; GMO; colorants; added chemicals, to address food deficiencies, and many other substances designed to enhance shelf life and maximize profit for a handful of companies. You should focus on cooking only organic, locally grown, wholesome food that you understand where they came from. If you cannot follow a product's history, or if these products were processed, you should avoid them at all costs. Train your taste to learn to love nutritional food. Minimize and or avoid the consumption of modern meats. Although prehistorical man is known to have been partially raised on a meat diet, the meat of today's modern society is not the same as the free-range animals that our ancestors ate. Our meat today is created in concentrated animal feeding operation (CAFO) or animal feeding operation (AFO). Here, over 1000 animal units are confined for over 45 days a year. These conditions, when the animals have very limited amount of mobility, promote diseases and unsanitary conditions, as animals in many instances are standing on their own manure. CAFO conditions then necessitate the use of antibiotics to keep these animals from getting sick. According to the FDA, up to 80 percent of all the antibiotics sold are used in food-producing farm animals. When we eat these animals, we consume this vast quantity of antibiotics — estimated to be more than 200,000 tons by 2030. In addition to the consumption of the antibiotics that animals eat, one is also consuming the hormones that these animals are fed to increase their size and optimize the profits. If one must eat highly industrialized meat, one needs to keep it to just a few ounces per week. Instead of red and white meat, one should switch to fish and marine animals that are wild-caught and toxins free. Although these may contain mercury and other toxins found in the oceans, in general, they are less dangerous than the cow, chicken, pork, and dairy (by-products) found in the typical American diets.

Research has widely documented the effects of a plant-based diet. All nutrients needed by the body can be readily obtained from plants. Our ancestors were plant-eaters, as meat was not so easy to hunt. The consumption of a moderate amount of meat, coupled with a healthy portion of fruits, vegetables, legumes, probiotics, prebiotics, and plant-based phytonutrients, is the optimum eating habit for holistic, fit individuals. Exercise and meditation will complement this good eating habit to produce the Efenian-minded self.

Food is the only medicine that the body needs: The primary function of food is to provide all the nutrients that the body needs to function optimally. This food depends on your living environment, as the body is highly adaptable: it changes and adapts to any type of condition. When adding too much of any one type of nutrient, or when we lack the nutrient needed altogether, then the body breaks down and diseases occur. Organic, natural whole foods from the local environments are all that is required to keep a healthy body and mind. When the body is fueled by a complete diet, it becomes more resilient. Chronic inflammation is a major factor in several maladies like diabetes, obesity, lung diseases, and heart disease, and nervous system diseases. A diet rich in fruits, vegetables, legumes, fiber, spices, and probiotics has been shown to suppress chronic inflammation and maladies. On the contrary, a diet of processed foods, sugars, and processed fats can trigger obesity, diabetes and, in general, leave us tired and craving for more food. Nutrition is ecosystem-driven food. The food required by the body is related to your living environment. Like most animals, we live in an ecosystem that produces epigenetic changes in our body and causes us to optimize our systems to the available food for the environment. Our requirements are more varied as, unlike most animals, the human-animal is highly mobile and lives in any many types of ecosystems. Nature uses time to optimize chemicals, systems, and processes. Natural nutrients feed the body and soul.

Microbiome—the second brain

One neglected part of holistic health is the microbiome – the collection of microbes that lives in our bodies and on our skin— the flora of microorganisms that lives within us and is an integral part of the human being. We are 90 percent microbial, which means that the portion of us we consider the "human" is actually a small part of the entire biological body. There are over 10 trillion microbes that inhabit the human body and most of them live in the gut and intestines, where they help us digest food, synthesize vitamins, and fight off infections. This entire ecosystem of bacteria and vast neural network – more than 100 million neurons – operating in our guts is being called our second brain. As such, one should re-evaluate what it means to be human when we are mostly microbes. These microorganisms are vital to our existence and wellbeing. Research evidence suggests that the gut microbiota may be at the heart of everything, being implicated in virtually all physiological or pathological situations. Gut microbiota has been implicated in the maturation and modulation of the host immune response, interactions – positive or negative – with pathogens, regulation of bone density, vitamin biosynthesis, and even daily host energy requirements. Considering all these influences, one can understand why the microbiome is associated with a plethora of conditions, ranging from obesity to cardiovascular diseases, chronic inflammatory diseases, and cancer.

When considering how to best feed and take care of our body, the microbiome must be a part of the consideration. In his book, *The Human Superorganism*, Rodney Dietert describes at length the role of the microbiome in the body: its immune system connection, and its overall influential interaction with the environment and with all external factors we face daily. One of his main arguments is that the microbiome is the arbiter of immune system homeostasis. He argues that the microbiome affects all aspects of our health, from food allergies to depression. Factors like the overuse of antibiotics, the crowed living conditions of city living, the current medical system of just treating symptoms and not treating the real cause of maladies, the food revolution – fast-food and the calorie-rich, nutrient-deprived food we eat— —all contribute to the depletion of beneficial bacteria in the microbiome, thus resulting in maladies. Food diversity is also another factor contributing to the killing of the good bacteria in our microbiome. Additionally, he argues that "rebiosis" — re-seeding the body with good bacteria — is a feasible way, no matter your age, toward a healthy microbiome, and this process may, in turn, usher a new era of individualized health care resulting in a dramatic reduction of Non-communicable Diseases (NCD's). In spite of all our technological advantages, we have found ourselves with more than 65 percent of deaths being caused by NCDs. These include heart diseases, diabetes, osteoarthritis, celiac diseases, psoriasis, and several others. The number of chronic illnesses continues to skyrocket, and there is a direct correction between this and the deterioration of the microbiome.

Rodney points out that there is good news, as we can revert this trend by focusing on rebiosis and changing our lifestyle to a more microbiome friendly one. The concept to truly own is that we are a combination of good bacteria — microorganisms — and human cells; one cannot exist without each other. Hence, we need to consider this whole human superorganism as one, and feed it, maintain it, and nurture it as one. Microbes are not our enemies; they are an integral part of us. When we operate with a mentality that we must over sanitize everything, kill every virus and bacteria and, in general, view these as our foes, we will continue the spiked illness trend. By changing our mindset to one that embraces this concept and by doing the beneficial changes needed to maintain this superorganism, then and only then can we make progress towards holistic health.

Detoxing is about getting your body back to harmony with nature: The body is constantly being exposed to toxins. Toxins are any chemical in large enough dosage to cause harm to the body. Heavy metals, preservatives, pesticides, insecticides, radiation, antibiotics, some water, some vaccines, etc., are all sources of toxins. Toxins kill the microbiome which, in turn, results in the above-mentioned maladies.

CHAPTER 11: ABSTEMIOUSNESS – LIFE'S GIFT

ON THE HEALING POWERS OF FASTING

The light of the world will illuminate within you when you fast and purify yourself.

— Mahatma Gandhi

T he willing abstinence of food—fasting—has as much beneficial effect on the body as its mortal enemy, feeding. The ancient practice of fasting has been used by all major religious leaders like Jesus, Muhammad, and Buddha. If you are a Christian, Jewish, Muslim, Buddhist, Hindu, Rastafarian, or Mormon, you are highly likely familiar with the practicing of fasting. Hippocrates, the father of Western medicine, believed fasting enables the body to heal itself.

"Everyone has a doctor in him; we just have to help him in his work.

The NATURAL *healing force within each one of us is the greatest force*

in getting well ...to eat when you are sick, is to feed your sickness."

— *Hippocrates*

Fasting has been scientifically proven to promote health by reducing or eliminating obesity, reducing inflammation, improving heart health, boosting brain function, preventing neurodegenerative disorders, improving metabolism, increasing growth hormones, delaying aging, and aiding in cancer prevention.

Fasting—a tale of ameliorations

Fasting heals and grows the body. In *The Obesity Code – Unlocking the Secret of Weight Loss,* Jason Fung and Tim Noakes describe in detail the scientific proof of the benefits of fasting. They argue that fasting can help you eliminate Type II diabetics, improve overall health, slow down aging—by reducing excess skin and signs of wear and tear—and optimize your metabolism. The mechanism of fasting is reducing body fat by eliminating the overproduction of insulin—eliminating or reducing insulin resistance—and by forcing the body to use the stored fat as the primary source of energy. By reducing your fat, you will also improve your muscle definition, size, and effectiveness of most organs and tissues: if they do not have to deal with the excess layer of fat, the muscles and other tissues can focus more on doing what they were designed to do.

Jason and Noakes argue that excess calories are not the real cause of obesity. They suggest that obesity is a hormonal imbalance caused by our toxic foods and environments, and by our bad habits of eating frequent snacks and consuming often way too much of the abundant processed foods, refined carbs, and added sugars. These have the effect of maintaining an elevated insulin level on a very consistent basis, which prevents the body from using fat as fuel and, instead, promotes fat storage. This is exacerbated by the high stress typical of our modern society, as well as lack of physical activities, which all eventually lead to the obese body, to developing insulin resistance, and to the onset of diabetes.

The cause of the current epidemic of obesity can be attributed to a constant state of insulin production by the body brought about by the constant supply of food in our modern society. When we eat food, insulin is produced to mobilize this energy to different parts of the body. Energy that is not needed is stored as glycogen — short-term energy reserves in muscles and liver — and the rest as fat. Several hours later, as the glucose level drops, glycogen reserves are used for energy. Once all glycogen is used up, then and only then will the body start breaking down fat stores for energy. As we are encouraged to eat every few hours, we never reach a state when we are depleted of energy and require the additional, stored fat. It is this constant feeding, with the aid of insulin, that is producing the obese state of modern societies. We have been told breakfast is the important meal of the day — without any research backing up this claim — and we are encouraged to snack every time hunger shows up. To control obesity, Jason and Noakes suggest using intermittent fasting on a regular basis and, when feeding, to eat whole, unprocessed plant-based foods that trigger only a small or minimal insulin response. Foods to be included are plenty of vegetables, legumes, fruits, and unprocessed fats — such as olive oils and butter. They argue for eating to reset and balance insulin in the body.

On the physiology of fasting

Fasting improves your immune system. As the body gets "lean" by reducing your body fat composition, it also becomes more effective. The effectiveness of the body causes your muscles and metabolism to work in a more efficient manner which, in turn, grows and makes your immune system cells grow and become more resistant to pathogens — stronger immune system. There is evidence that suggests that interval fasting may prolong life span. A study published in the *American Journal of Clinical Nutrition* investigated whether alternate-day fasting is a feasible method of dietary restriction in nonobese humans, and whether it improves known biomarkers of longevity. The study included nonobese subjects, eight men and eight women, who fasted every other day for twenty-two days. Several biomarkers were baselined and then measured at some prescribed intervals. The markers included body weight, body composition, resting metabolic rate (RMR), respiratory quotient (RQ), temperature, fasting serum glucose, insulin, free fatty acids, and ghrelin. Researchers found that subjects lost an average of 2.5 lbs. RMR and RQ did not change significantly from baseline. Glucose and ghrelin did not change significantly from baseline, whereas fasting insulin decreased 57 percent. The authors concluded that alternate-day fasting was feasible in nonobese subjects and fat oxidation increased. The leading parameter in any fasting regime is the reduction of overproduction of insulin, due to the constant feeding, and its associated consequences. Insulin is a critical hormone of an optimum performing body. It regulates blood glucose, and it is involved in how the fat is used by the body. Insulin signals fat cells to take up glucose to store as triglycerides. An additional effect of insulin is in inhibiting the breakdown of fats. It is this function that gets disrupted by fasting. By not having insulin in the body, the body is forced to use the fat reserves, thus reducing the overall body fat percent.

Everybody responds differently to fasting, as each body is unique in composition and microbiome. Considering this fact, it is advised that anyone considering a fasting plan consults a medical professional to ensure proper execution and to avoid any potential complications. This narrative is a mere compilation of scientific studies to assist you in making an informed decision and it is in no way meant as a medical recommendation.

What exactly is happening inside our bodies when we fast? Henry woke up to the disturbing alarm that annoyingly pushes him out of bed by 5:30 am every weekday. This morning was uneventful, except for the fact that today he was going to start his fasting program. He was going to observe, feel, and sense carefully how his body was going to react to the experience. He did stay out the night before beyond the regular sleeping time that he self-polices to ensure he gets at least seven hours of sleep. At the onset of his program—in the first three hours—his obese body is still digesting the hamburger, chips, and beers he hastily ate during the football game before going to sleep. His body broke down all the carbohydrates, protein, and fat of his eating feast into glucose, amino acids, fatty acids, all destined to be used for energy or to be stored for later use. This heavy carbs-loaded meal produced a high level of glucose in the bloodstream, which triggered the pancreas to secrete insulin. Insulin moves the glucose into cells where it can be used for energy production, protein synthesis, or store as glycogen—short-term storage of glucose—or as adipose tissue, fat—long-term storage. At this stage, Henry is in an anabolic state as nutrients are available for growth. By the end of his first three-hour interval, his glucose and insulin levels are likely back to his pre-meal markers. During this time, Henry is also feeling swings of hunger and satiety, due to signals driven by changes in ghrelin—the hunger hormone, which turns on appetite—and leptin—which suppresses appetite.

After four hours of no food consumption, Henry's body starts entering the catabolic stage—a breakdown of molecules into smaller units that are oxidized or used in other anabolic reactions. The body is extremely smart in its response to energy demands from any of its constituents. As the blood glucose level drops, glucagon—the opposite hormone of insulin—stimulates the breakdown, catabolic function, of glycogen for energy. Glycogen is the main source of energy for the body. This process will continue as needed to ensure enough glucose is available. Henry, committed to his fasting, is not adding any nutrients to his body other than water. As the hours in his plan advance, he starts to deplete his glycogen stores. The necessity for fuel is constant; thus, his body starts to look for alternative forms of energy. His body—with glucose reserves nearly gone—changes the course of energy supply from glucose to fats and ketone reserves. Exactly when this change happens, he could not tell. Considering how much fuel he consumed prior to the beginning of fasting, this change happened likely later rather than sooner. Sixteen hours into his fasting, Henry's body is going into the fat-burning mode via a process called lipolysis—the breakdown of fat into free fatty acids.

Fatty acids in the liver are then transformed into ketones, ketosis via a process called beta-oxidation. The process of ketosis is now burning Henry's fat for energy, due to a lack of glycogen stores. Once ketosis starts, ketones become the primary fuel. The brain still requires some glucose, although it prefers ketones as energy sources. His body can produce glucose, sugar, from non-carbohydrate sources like fat, ketones, amino acids, and proteins, via a process referred to as gluconeogenesis. Several studies have shown the benefits of being in ketosis beyond the main one of losing weight. Ketones are a much cleaner fuel for the body; they are a consistent form of fuel as oppose to the spike of typical carbs. The brain needs a consistent energy source and ketones, when present, seem to be this ideal source; furthermore, they lead to better mental focus. Studies also have shown that cancer cells feed off sugar; however, these cells do not use ketones as fuel. Consequently, being in ketosis often deprives cancer cells of their food source.

Henry's third day of fasting has arrived, loaded with discipline and painful absolute resolutions. His body is now on a prolonged fasting phase. Fasting reduces the number of inputs the digestive system needs to break down and reassemble. The pancreas, stomach, gall bladder, liver, and intestine, all get to rest while fasting — a sabbath for your insides — and resting is very restorative. Glucose and insulin levels are extremely low, and hunger is now suppressed; his body is in a steady state of ketosis. IGF-1, the insulin-like growth factor, is decreased by the liver. IGF-1 is a hormone responsible for growth and development. This decrease has been associated with a less oxidative stress and may take part in reducing some form of cancers and having some anti-aging effects. Prolonged fasting has also been shown to activate resistance to toxins.

It is worth mentioning a dangerous condition, ketoacidosis, sometimes associated with diabetes and long term fasting. This condition is not to be confused with ketosis. Diabetic ketoacidosis, DKA, dangerously acidic blood from overly high ketone levels, usually only seen in alcoholics, diabetics, and cases of extreme starvation, is a severe and life-threatening complication. DKA occurs when the cells in our body do not receive the sugar, glucose, they need for energy. This happens when there is enough glucose in the bloodstream, but not enough insulin to help convert glucose for use in the cells. The body, realizing this event, starts breaking down muscle and fat for energy. This breakdown produces ketones which cause an imbalance in the electrolyte system leading to ketoacidosis. Normal insulin production typically tells the body to stop increasing its production of ketones and then these plateau at a safe level; however, since insulin levels are low for a long time during extreme fasting, this feedback loop does not occur. Typical symptoms of DKA include dry skin, abdominal pain, shortness of breath, deep rapid breathing, nausea, and dehydration.

Hungering universal sustenance

A great number of studies have shown that Intermittent fasting (IF) has powerful benefits for the body and the brain. This practice was very common for our ancestors throughout human evolution. Refrigeration and supermarkets are a very recent innovation. Our ancestors did not have the luxury of storing food, thus they ate what they caught and sometimes, when food was scarce, they would go for days without consuming any food. Humans evolved to be able to function without food for extended periods of time. IF is an eating pattern consisting of cycles of eating and fasting. One of the most common patterns is the 16/8 — This entails 16 hours of fasting and an 8-hour eating window and done at least twice a week. This is a popular pattern because, when combined with the sleeping cycles — sleep for eight hours — then only eight hours of fasting are needed. For example, a person stops eating at 8:00 pm, then sixteen hours later — sleeping hours included — he would start eating again at 12:00 noon. This cycle is relatively simple to implement and easily kept for the long term. The IF cycles are not concerned with the specific foods consumed, but with the interval of time when the food is eaten. However, for optimum benefit from this procedure, a proper plant-based and complete diet must be maintained. IF does not only help with weight management, but it also boosts metabolism which assists in keeping the weight down and the energy level high.

The benefits of IF are many. A study done by the University of Aberdeen Rowett Institute of Nutrition and Health found that IF is an option for achieving weight loss and maintenance. Many of the people using IF do so with the hope of losing weight and reducing overall fat content, belly fat, and waist circumference. Studies show that people lose 4-7 percent of their waist circumference when involved in IF practice. Due to the nature of the small window allowed in IF, subjects end up eating fewer meals and consuming fewer calories. Weight loss is additionally stimulated as IF enhances hormone functions. The lower level of insulin, higher levels of growth hormones, and increased amounts of norepinephrine resulting from IF increase the breakdown of fat and facilitate its use for energy in the body. Short-term fasting increases your metabolic rate by 3.6 to 14%, helping in burning more calories. Intermittent fasting works on two modalities to assist in weight management: calorie reduction and metabolism increase. It can cause significant weight loss of 3-8% over 3-24 weeks.

Intermittent fasting has also been shown to prevent insulin resistance – the main cause of diabetes – and to reduce blood sugar levels. Studies have shown fasting insulin has been reduced by 20-31 percent, and blood sugar by 3-6 percent. A study in diabetic rats also showed that intermittent fasting protected against kidney damage, one of the most severe complications of diabetes. With diabetes at an epidemic level in the United States, IF seem to provide a ray hope in the dizzying selection of fast and highly processed food options.

Free radicals from oxidative stress and chronic inflammation are two leading causes of premature aging, body deterioration, and several chronic maladies. Studies have found IF can reduce oxidative stress and inflammation in the body. Free radicals are unstable molecules looking to react with other molecules, like DNA, and by so doing they damage these molecules in the process. IF may have benefits against aging and the development of numerous diseases. Intermittent fasting has also been shown to improve several risk factors of heart diseases like blood pressure, cholesterol, triglycerides, and blood sugar and inflammatory markers. In animal models, IF has additionally been proven to prevent cancers.

Cells in the body go through a process called autophagy. This is the way the body has of cleaning out damaged cells in order to regenerate newer, healthier cells. This is in an anti-aging principle, a kind of turning back the clock and creating younger cells. When we fast, the cells in the body initiate this process of autophagy. The body keeps breaking down cellular material and reusing it for necessary processes; this is a kind of waste removal process. IF triggers the metabolic pathway of autophagy to remove waste material from cells. One of the most significant benefits of IF is its effect on brain health.

Befogged brain no longer—fasting brings the light

Intermittent fasting has been found to improve various metabolic features known to be critical to brain health. Studies in rats have shown an increase in the growth of new nerve cells by using IF which benefits the brain. It also increased the level of brain-derived neurotrophic factor (BDNF), a deficiency of which has been related to depression and several other brain issues. Additionally, animal studies have also shown that IF protects against brain damage due to strokes. The benefits of IF to brain functions are many. It may, as well, increase the growth of new neurons and protect the brain from damage.

Alzheimer's disease is one of the most common neurodegenerative diseases in the world. IF may help prevent Alzheimer's disease. With no cure in sight for Alzheimer's, prevention is our current best choice. An animal study on rats showed that IF may delay the onset of Alzheimer's disease or reduce its severity. In a series of reports, an intervention that included daily short-term fasts was able to significantly improve Alzheimer's symptoms in 9 out of 10 subjects studied. Animal studies also point to IF being able to protect against several other neurodegenerative diseases like Parkinson's and Huntington's disease. Researchers have concluded that IF regimens can ameliorate age-related deficits in cognitive functions.

One of the most promising benefits of IF is that it may extend the human lifespan. Studies in rats have shown that IF extends the lifespan of rats by as much as 83 percent longer than those rats that did not fast. Although this does not mean a direct translation into humans, it points to the possibility of lifespan improvement in humans. Given all the above benefits of IF, it follows that intermittent fasting could help tremendously to a longer and healthier life.

Mental tranquility is also an effect of fasting: Fasting has been practiced by virtually every major religion as a form of penance, sacrifice, and or sign of faith. Jesus was said to fast for four days and forty nights, Muslims observe Ramadan—a month of daytime fasting—and many other religions have variations on this practice. This practice has a calming effect on the mind and produces an overall positive outlook as the benefits become more and more visible.

PART FIVE: THE FIFTH NOBLE TRUTH

Body in Motion is Thy Path

Eppur si muove – and yet it moves

— Galileo Galilei

In 1616, the Catholic Church placed Nicholas Copernicus's book, *De Revolutionibus* – the first scientific argument for a heliocentric (sun-centered) universe – on its list of banned books. In 1632, Galileo published his *Dialogue Concerning the Two Chief World Systems* in which he argued both sides of the heliocentrism debate. His position on the debate was clear as he understood the sun was the center, not the earth. He named the arguments in favor of geocentrism – "Simplicius" – which implied his favored side of the arguments

.

Using Simplicius—simpleton—for the geocentrism argument did not buy him any favor with the Church either. Pope Paul V summoned Galileo to Rome to tell him he could no longer support Copernicus publicly. In 1633, he was summoned before the Roman inquisition. Initially, he denied that he supported heliocentrism, but later he said he had only done so unintentionally. The Church asked him to recant his public statements that the earth moves around the sun and not the other way around. The Church's scripture said that, since the sun stood still in the sky to prolong a day of victorious battle at a given point in the Old Testament, it ipso facto had to circle the earth. Galileo's statements that the earth was a sphere rotating on its own axis, and orbiting around the sun, had defamed Church teaching. After being forced during his trail to admit that the earth was the stationary center of the universe, Galileo allegedly muttered *Eppur si muove*—*And yet it moves*. Galileo was convicted of "vehement suspicion of heresy" and under threat of torture was forced to express sorrow and curse his errors.

Galileo Galilei (1564-1642) was obsessed with the motion of heavenly bodies. He is regarded as the father of modern science, and his contribution expands the realm of physics, astronomy, mathematics, philosophy, and cosmology. He was born in Pisa, Italy, in 1564, the first of six children of Vincenzo Galilei—a musician and scholar. Vincenzo wanted his firstborn son to become a physician, so he named his child after his ancestor, Galileo Bonaiuti, who was a well-known physician. At age sixteen, young Galileo enrolled at the University of Pisa where he was going to study medicine but was quickly sidetracked to mathematics. Galileo always performed his best academically, even though he did not find much pleasure in doing so. During his years at the University of Pisa, he was forced to live in a small house with his uncle. He would be looked down upon by students and professors based, in part, on his raggedy appearance. His father struggled to send him to school as they were extremely limited in financial resources. He studied rather hard during those years in his area of interest—mathematics—but he left the University of Pisa in 1585 without a diploma. At age twenty-five, he was still living with his parents with no job or money to go back to the university. His father had become discouraged, and his mother often called him lazy.

Galileo returned to the University of Pisa to teach mathematics after getting an invitation from the Grand Duke, Ferdinand Medici of Tuscany. It was during this period as a professor that he was credited with the discovery of the law of falling bodies – his most significant contribution to physics. From 1589 to 1610, he was chair of mathematics at the universities of Pisa and then Padua. During one of his frequent trips to Venice, he met a young woman named Marina Gamba, daughter of Andrea Gamba. They began a romantic relationship. She moved into his house in Padua and together they had three children out of wedlock: Virginia – later Sister Maria Celeste; Livia – later Sister Arcangela; and Vincenzo. Not in any of their baptismal records is the father's name, Galileo, mentioned. Virginia was described as "daughter by fornication of Marina of Venice." Livia's baptismal had a blank line where the father's name was expected. Vincenzo's baptismal record announced, "father uncertain." Because of his professor position and his friendships with Venetian nobility, it would have been unwise for him to appear as the children's father. In 1610, he left Padua and took a position at the royal court of the Medici family in Florence. His two daughters accompanied him, but his 4-year-old son Vincenzo was left with Marina. Vincenzo would eventually end up joining him in Florence a few years later. With Marina out of the picture, Galileo enrolled his daughters in a convent and had Vincenzo legitimated by the Grand Duke of Tuscany. Due to the illegitimate nature of his daughters, Galileo believed that the girls would be unmarriageable. Their only alternative was religious life. Both girls were accepted into the San Matteo convent, where they remained for the rest of their lives. Vincenzo studied law and later became a lutenist like his grandfather.

Galileo made countless contributions to science during his time. When thinking of bodies in motion, the name Galileo bubbles out. Galileo's laws of motion – which came about from his measurements that all bodies accelerate at the same rate regardless of their mass or size – paved the way for the theories of classical mechanics by Isaac Newton. His heliocentric theories, with modification by Kepler, became accepted as scientific facts. Galileo invented an improved telescope that allowed him to discover craters and mountains on the moon, the phases of Venus, Jupiter's moons, and the stars of the Milky Way. 1n 1583, he discovered the rules that govern the motion of pendulums, thus transforming how time was to be measured. According to Stephen Hawking, Galileo probably bears more of the responsibility for the birth of modern science than anybody else. Albert Einstein called him the father of modern science.

After his trials with the Roman inquisition, 70-year-old Galileo lived his last seven years under comfortable house arrest. He used this time to write a summary for his early motion experiments that later became his final great scientific work — *Two New Sciences*. He died in Arcetri, near Florence, at the age of 77, after suffering from heart palpitations and fever. In 1744, Galileo's *Dialogue* was removed from the Church's list of banned books, and in the 20th century, Popes Pius XII and John Paul II made official statements of regret for how the Church had treated Galileo. He brilliantly studied and described all types of bodies' motions. Motion in science is referred to as a change with time in the position or orientation of a body. Everything experiences motion, not a single matter — even the most fundamental ones — Quartz and Leptons — can escape motion. Life itself is a result of motion, as energy in motion is organized and packed in atoms and molecules, and eventually complex biological creatures. The electron, a fundamental part of every atom, is nothing but rotating energy, energy in motion. Albert Einstein's famous equation, $E=MC^2$, connects the motion of matter to its energy. Without motion, life is impossible. Total equilibrium is death. We must keep moving, constantly challenging our physical bodies. Modern society calls this motion of the human body, exercise. If one is creating enough motion in our bodies of enough intensity to make it sweat, and including all 650 muscles of the body, one is nurturing life and promoting health. Keeping the body moving most of the time, one finds a balance between motion and stillness, and one gets rewarded with holistic fitness. Exercise, body in motion, is the key to maintaining the body in optimum physical shape and performance.

Chapter 12: My New Shiny Exoskeleton

SIX PACK — SWEAT FORGED

Good things come to those who sweat.

— Anonymous

Homo sapiens are naturally born runners. It is as if we were born to run. Our early ancestors were not endowed with any particularly impressive set of defense weapons against regular predators. They did not possess fangs, sharp claws, toxic poisons, powerful limbs or jaws, or any of the other key weapons of the animal kingdom; however, they had the key advantage of a highly superior brain which allowed them to use tools and solve predation problems more efficiently than any other animal on the planet. One can argue that the dexterity of their hands, their adroit skills, and their relatively strong limbs offer some physical advantages over some smaller predators. However, one key survival skill was their fast legs and their ability to run away from danger. Running was an early survival skill for our ancestors. The endurance running

179

hypothesis states that the evolution of certain human characteristics can be explained as adaptations to long-distance running. This hypothesis suggests that endurance running played an important role in early hominins in obtaining food. Researchers have proposed that this endurance began as an adaptation for scavenging and later for persistence hunting — persistence hunting is a form of pursuit hunting in which the hunter uses endurance running during the midday heat to drive prey into hyperthermia and exhaustion so they can easily be killed. Homo Sapiens is the only primate species that use this hunting technique. Humans have little hair, and their ability to sweat — an effective means of cooling the body — makes them superiorly adapted for endurance running. This technique is believed to have been used by early humans, and it is still in use by the Bushmen, Saan peoples, of the Kalahari Desert.

The fit individual was able to survive the early, sometimes harsh environment of early man. This need to be fit was a natural necessity to survive, and it was part of their natural daily habits and culture. In early humans, their physical conditions were developed through the physical demands of hunting, foraging, adaptable movement skills, and the innate instinct to survive. The modern version of physical fitness is more of a recent innovation. A healthy fit body is a muscular body, with a strong immune system, and highly functional metabolism. Muscles are sprouted by cultivating discipline-exercise. Muscles provide the source of movement for the body. In order to move optimally through your environment, you need a well-defined muscular structure. The large and well-built muscular structure increases your ability to survive, reproduce, and preserve the species. Survival of the fittest, in our modern-man interpretation, refers to the one with the highest advantages being able to survive the easiest. In this context, we are referring to fighting diseases and dangerous situations. Muscles will give the advantage needed to ensure optimal living. In general, fitness means different things to different people. The important take-home message is that embarking on any regular exercise will be of benefit to your health. The more exercise that is carried out, the healthier an individual will look and feel — including mental health and clarity, as well.

MY NEW SHINY EXOSKELETON

If we could give every individual the right amount of nourishment and exercise, not too little and not too much, we would have found the safest way to health.

— Hippocrates

Ontology of motion

Our ancestors had to be physically fit, or the alternative was to become dinner for a hungry predator. Although Darwin did not mean survival of the fittest as the "physical" fit, this does still make sense when applied to our early man — the physical fit survived and the weak perished. Hominids survived on hunting and gathering. These were very physically demanding activities, so our early ancestors were in great physical condition, just as wild animals are in today's environment. Wild animals need to be able to gather, and some need to kill their food — a condition that necessitates their best physical condition for their given habitat. Throughout most of human history, humans have needed to stay physically and competitively fit. This is a sharp contrast to today's society where the need for fitness is only a matter of reproductive desire. The modern man has no need to gather, hunt, or fight for his food; it is readily available at the nearest supermarket. This difference between our evolutionary fitness and our current state of fitness has great implications for the causation of maladies and overall mental health states. Studies of tribes who are still living close to the lifestyles of our ancestors show relatively fewer chronic. They also are leaner, have better physical conditioning, better natural diets, and more efficient metabolism. Mobility and physical activities are a regular part of these cultures.

Physical activity is more of an all-encompassing activity, and it refers to the expenditures of energy by body movements via the skeletal muscles. Exercise, on the other hand, is a subset of physical activity, and it refers to any training of the body to improve its function and enhance its fitness. Physical conditioning refers to the development of physical fitness by the adaptation of the body and its systems to an exercise program. In Western culture, the origin of physical culture is dated to the ancient Greeks. The first Olympics is traditionally dated to 776 BC. The ancient Olympic Games were originally a festival for Zeus. Early events included a wide range of physical contests – applicable to both sport and war – including foot races, javelin contests, and later wrestling. They held them in honor of Zeus and gave these mythological origins. The games were held every four years or Olympiad, and this became the standard time for modern Olympic games. The greatest Greek athlete of this time was Milo of Croton. He enjoyed a magnificent career in wrestling and won many victories in ancient Greece. He popularized progressive resistance training by carrying a calf daily from its birth until it became full-size. Milo was said to have carried a bull on his shoulders, and to have burst a band about his brow by simply inflating the veins of his temples. He was a six-time Olympic victor. He also won seven crowns at Pythian Games and nine at the Nemean Games. His career spanned over 24 years. Milo was said to consumed raw bull's meat and to drink its blood in front of his adversary, to create intimidation and fear in his competitors.

Physical culture for sports, as well as for war, was typical of most of the early civilized populations. Early sports were based on practical and natural motions related to readiness for war. As the industrial revolution rolled in, around 1760, there was a great transition from manual process to machine-based manufacturing process. As people became more sedentary, the move towards physical exercise was more prevalent and intentional. The move towards a better fit body through exercise was being made a source of national pride in many European countries. Being fit, healthy, and ready to serve at war was to become a civic duty.

The 21st century found a population that still values exercise and physical activity — — as a mean towards a healthy body; however, the excessive number of conveniences in all levels of affairs, the abundance of calorie-rich nutrient-deficient food, and the natural tendency of systems to preserve energy, all conspire to keep the modern human from being the best healthy self they can be. There is a consensus on the importance of regular exercise, and today nearly every neighborhood has a gym or place to work out. Yet, despite the plethora of resources for exercise, the average individual has never been so physically sedentary and out of shape. A recent World Health Organization report indicates that life expectancy in the United States has dropped for the first time since 1993. Despite our modern advances in medical technologies, the health of the modern man is declining.

Transformation by motion

The body of research on exercise and its benefits to the body is extensive. One can literally transform one's body performance and health using regular exercise. Exercise can improve nearly every aspect of health. It is the first line of defense to prevent and manage all types of chronic maladies. Regular physical activities can increase the production of hormones that make you feel happier and sleep better. It can also improve skin's appearance, help one lose weight, lessen the risk of chronic diseases, and improve sex life. According to a US Department of Health and Human Services report on physical activity, regular exercise significantly reduced the causes of mortality by up to 30% for men and women. These rates are consistent across all age groups and racial categories. The Center for Disease Control and Prevention (CDC) recommends 30 minutes of moderate to high-intensity exercise for a least five days a week for all healthy individuals.

Exercise, coupled with proper nutrition, is the key to fit bodies, and it helps maintain the optimum ratio of body fat. Weight is not a good metric of a fit body; a better metric to gauge physical health is core abdominal definition—" six-pack." A well-defined abdominal core muscle structure does not only make the body look great in appearance but is a great indicator of overall physical conditioning. Visceral fat—fat around the stomach area—is the hardest fat to get rid of as it is the preferred location for excess fat. If one is able to rid this area of excess fat, then it follows other areas that will be fat-free as well. A single-digit fat percent ratio is typically needed to obtain the six-packed visible muscles for men. A heavy individual could be in great physical fitness if she keeps a low enough body fat ratio.

Studies show that inactivity is a major factor in weight gain and obesity. While a calorie-deficit diet results in a lower metabolic rate, exercise has been shown to increase the metabolic rate, which aids in the burning of additional calories and helps to lose weight and fat. When one combines aerobic exercise with resistance training, one maximizes fat loss and muscle growth. A fast metabolism, aided by exercise, is then crucial to help maintain and grow muscle mass and reduce body fat percentage.

Exercise does not only grow the muscles, but it grows the bones as well. The physical activity associated with exercising stimulates muscle building by helping release hormones that promote the ability of muscles to absorb amino acids. These amino acids help the muscles grow and reduce their breakdown. Older people tend to lose muscle mass as they age; regular exercise is vital to reduce muscle loss and keep strength and fitness at any age. Exercise also helps prevent osteoporosis later in life. Studies have shown that high-impact exercises like running, soccer, and other impact sports promote higher bone density than low or non-impact exercises like swimming and cycling.

Exercise—driven muscularity—strong immune system

A study published in the US National Library of Medicine on low and moderate exercise training showed six weeks of regular exercise reduced levels of fatigue in a healthy, sedentary, sampled population who had reported persistent fatigue. Energy usage and metabolism in the body are closely related to the level of physical activity. A regular program of exercise increases the energy level of individuals and also metabolism — which results in optimum energy management within the body. Exercise can also increase the energy levels of people suffering from chronic fatigue syndrome (CFS). Furthermore, other studies have shown that exercise can increase energy levels in people suffering from progressive illness, such as cancer, HIV and multiple sclerosis.

Exercise has been found to strengthen the immune system. It promotes good blood circulation, which in turn allows the cells and substances of the immune system to move through the body freely and do their job more efficiently. Exercise slows down the release of stress hormones, thereby reducing the risk of maladies and easing the burden on the immune system. A strong immune system is the hallmark of fit individuals. By being able to fend off maladies, or by minimizing their cycle time when they occur, one can improve longevity and vitality. The improvement in strength, stamina, muscularity, and flexibility associated with a regular workout program all work together to optimize the ability of the body to fight off pathogens and, in general, survive better than the alternative option of not exercising.

Research shows that many of the negative changes associated with aging are actually caused by a lack of physical activity. A research study at the University of Texas Southwestern Medical School analyzed the physiological changes of five healthy volunteers. These individuals were asked to spend three weeks of the summer resting in bed. Testing the men before and after exercise, the researcher found disturbing changes that included faster resting heart rates, higher systolic blood pressures, a drop in the heart's maximum pumping capacity, a rise in body fat, and a fall in muscle strength. These changes in these mid-twenty's subjects were indicative of the detrimental effect of inactivity and lack of exercise. These young men show the physiological characteristics of men twice their age. The researchers continue their studies by putting their subjects on an 8-week exercise program. The program did much more than just reverse the deterioration caused by the bed rest, as some of the measurements were better than before they started the study. This study showed the harmful consequences of prolonged bed rest and inactivity. Many of the changes that physiologists attribute to aging are caused by disuse. Using the body will keep it young.

Oxidation and chronic inflammation are key processes of aging. Oxidation is a normal and necessary process that occurs in the body. However, oxidative stress happens when there's an imbalance between free radicals and antioxidants. If there are more free radicals present than can be kept in balance by antioxidants, the free radicals can start doing damage to fatty tissue, DNA, and proteins in your body. The body is mostly made of proteins, lipids, and DNA. This damage can result in aging and several chronic conditions. Inflation is a natural response of the immune system to pathogens. But when this condition is kept for a long time, becoming chronic inflammation, it becomes damaging to the body. Cortisol is the best anti-inflammatory hormone that the body makes, but prolonged exposure to these hormones results in deterioration of the body.

Exercise plays a role, also, in the sleeping patterns and quality of sleep of individuals. It can help you to fall asleep faster and additionally stay asleep longer. Sleeping is key to a fit and healthy body as it allows the body and mind to regenerate during this time and reboot all learned facts, and it is also believed that sleeping reinforces synapse connection, thus consolidating and verifying all the learned experiences of the day. One cannot function optimally without adequate sleep. Rest is as important as exercise.

Muscular physique is not only an image of sustained dedication and pride, but it also reflects the commitment that the individual has spent on their body. Individuals with a well-defined muscular composition are not only attractive to look at, but they are also a reminder of what physical health looks like. Studies have shown that lack of exercise is one of the major causes of most chronic maladies. Considerable evidence proves that reductions in daily physical activity are the primary cause of chronic conditions and that exercise is rehabilitative treatment from the lack of activity dysfunction. The lack of physical activity has been linked to 35 pathological and clinical conditions, like obesity, diabetes, liver diseases, cognitive functions and diseases, cardiovascular diseases, cancer, digestive tract diseases, pulmonary and kidney diseases, metabolic syndrome, bone and connective tissue disorders, and reproductive diseases. The body quickly adapts to insufficient physical activity, and when this is done routinely, it results in a substantial decrease in both total and quality years of life. Physical activity, on the other hand, not only prevents, or delays, chronic diseases, but also increases longevity. Exercise strengthens the heart and improves circulation, thus raising the oxygen levels in the body. Endurance athletes' hearts show expanded left and right ventricles, whereas strength athletes show thickening of their heart wall, especially their left ventricles. This lowers the risk of heart diseases and stabilizes blood pressure. Exercise can, additionally, lower triglycerides levels. Chronic diseases need not be a certain outcome of modern man — exercise can stop this trend. Physical activity is critical to maintaining a healthy weight and to reduce the onset of chronic diseases. A routine of regular exercise has been shown to improve cardiovascular fitness, body composition, and even to decrease blood pressure levels. Exercise also lowers blood sugar and insulin levels. This can cut down the risk of metabolic syndrome and type 2 diabetes. If these maladies are already present, then exercise can help better manage them.

Mind and body—divine duality

Several epidemiological studies have shown that exercise improves one's self-esteem and a sense of wellbeing. Age-related memory and cognitive functions have been shown to have slower rates when the individual is engaged in a regular exercise routine as compared to sedentary people. Adults who have a higher level of physical activity have fewer depressive and anxiety symptoms. This supports the idea that exercise offers a protective effect against the development of mental disorders. During exercise, the body releases chemicals that can improve moods, create a feel-good sensation, and give an overall feeling of relaxation. These help with stress-reducing and also reducing the risk of depression.

Neurogenesis — the process of creating new neurons using stem cells — has been found to be correlated to exercise activities. Physical activity impacts several biological, as well as psychological, mechanisms. For example, meta-analyses show that exercise reduces anxiety in clinical settings. Animal studies have shown exercise up-regulates hippocampal neurogenesis. New neuronal growth in the brain, especially in the hippocampus — the area of the brain related to verbal memory and learning — has been implicated in the treatment of psychiatric conditions, including depression and anxiety. A research study done at the University of British Columbia found that regular aerobic exercise appears to increase the size of the hippocampus. Brain fog is reduced and the ability to learn new information is improved when one exercises.

The mounting amount of evidence for exercise-derived brain benefits is not controversial in any sense. Many studies show a strong relationship between these two. One of the most abundant brain neurotrophins – these are families of proteins that induce the survival, development, and functions of neurons – is Brain-derived neurotrophic factor (BDNF). BDNF has been linked to both anxiety and depression. The reduced level of BDNF in the hippocampus has been correlated to stress-induced depressive and anxious behaviors. Increased levels of BDNF have been shown to have antidepressant effects. After physical activity, it has been observed that the level of BDNF is higher. This may suggest a mechanism for reducing anxiety and depression by practicing exercises routines. It has also been noticed that exercise promotes the production of neurotrophins, which lead to greater brain plasticity, better memory, and sharper learning ability. Additionally, exercise increases neurotransmitters in the brain, specifically serotonin and norepinephrine, both of which boost information processing and mood. Exercises practically increase the thickness of the cerebral cortex, thus improving brain functions.

Cases of dementia are on the rise. In fact, researchers have found that there is one new case of dementia, globally, every four seconds. Exercise helps both memory and thinking. Mechanisms by which exercise improves brain performance includes the reduction of insulin resistance, reduction of inflammation, and the stimulation of growth factor – these are chemicals in the brain responsible for the health of brain cells, the growth of new blood vessels in the brain, and the abundance and survival of new brain cells. Insulin resistance is linked to several diseases, but primarily diabetes. Chronic inflammation is very detrimental to the body. Exercise helps reduce or eliminate both conditions. Exercise improves mood, sleep, and reduces stress and anxiety. These are all implicated with cognitive impairment. Studies have additionally shown that people who exercise regularly have greater volume in the prefrontal cortex – the area of the brain responsible for thinking and memory – over those who do not exercise. Scott McGinnis, a neurologist at Brigham and Women's Hospital and professor of neurology at Harvard Medical School, says that, "Even more exciting is the finding that engaging in a program of regular exercise of moderate intensity over six months or a year is associated with an increase in the volume of selected brain regions." Exercise improves cognitive health in many different ways. When a person is engaged in aerobic exercise, their heart rate and blood flow are increased, and both of these increase the blood flow to the brain. The more the intensity of the workout, the more oxygen goes into the bloodstream, and more oxygen is delivered to the brain. This leads to neurogenesis which increases brain volume and helps against the effects of dementia. Exercise could potentially delay dementia onset by as much as 15 years.

Exercising can be a tool to help quit smoking. It makes it easier to quit smoking by reducing cravings and withdrawal symptoms. It could also limit the weight one may get when one stops smoking. Exercising has also an age-reducing component, as it can slow down the aging process. By promoting the growth of muscle, by improving brain functions, reducing stress, reducing disease occurrence, and generating a happier mood, exercise can extend one's overall mortality rate. Sexual health is also improved with exercise. A regular program of exercise may lower the risk of erectile dysfunction (ED) in men and, for those who already have it may improve their sexual function. In women, exercise may increase sexual arousal.

On exercising mechanics

Exercise is the only path to heal and grow the body. Body and mind act as one. But a strong mind needs a strong body. The only way to get a strong body is to get the body in motion, to get the body to do work, purposely intended exercise. This iterative process of working the muscle to exhaustion forces the muscle to grow and promotes the immune system to grow, as well, and consequently to become stronger. Exercise is the key to ultimate health. A successful workout routine has to include aerobic and anaerobic workouts. Strength workout, like lifting weights, is used to quickly build muscle size. Anaerobic is needed to keep the body power output high and to be able to deliver explosive response on demand. Training like running, boxing, or physical sports are great ways to get your anaerobic exercises. Intermittent fasting, when coupled with intermittent exercise maximizes fat loss. Intermittent exercise is when one goes as hard and as fast as one can, then one recovers for just a few seconds – 20 seconds or so – and then continues with the exercise until the routine is done. This form of exercise puts the maximum amount of stress on the body and ensures that you are sweating and working out your cardio endurance. When these two intermittent forms are used together, you get the maximum results.

Cardiorespiratory endurance refers to how the body can supply fuel during a physical activity using the circulatory system. Activities that raise the heart rate for a sustained period of time improve cardiorespiratory endurance. Examples of these activities are running, cycling, swimming. People that are regularly involved in these activities have a better physically fit body. It is critical to start any physical activity slowly and with the supervision of a medical professional. When the heart gets stronger via aerobic exercises, it delivers more blood and small arteries are made to grow within the tissues so that blood can reach the muscles more effectively. The American College of Sports Medicine recommends aerobic exercise 3-5 times per week for 30-60 minutes at 65-85 percent of the maximum heart rates.

Stretching is paramount in any exercise program to avoid injuries and maximize flexibility. Daily stretching helps the body improve its range of motion and "lubricate" the joints, thus avoiding premature degeneration of tissues. Flexibility is the range of movement across a joint. As the muscle gains flexibility, the likelihood of injuries is reduced dramatically, as the muscles are able to respond better to resistance and sudden moves during various activities. After a particularly hard workout, the muscles become tight; stretching in this situation helps relieve post-exercise aches and pains. A slow and well-executed stretching session improves blood circulation throughout the entire body and this, in turn, helps provide nutrients to the aching muscles and joints and promotes muscle relaxation and stress reduction. Flexibility is a key component of the Fitness Quotient due to its primal role for overall fitness. By increasing body flexibility, one improves body posture, mechanical efficiency, and overall functional performance. Flexible bodies have higher performance than stiff ones because they create more energy-efficient movements. A daily stretching regimen is the simplest and most efficient way of achieving whole-body flexibility. One technique used by high-performance athletes is using an ice bath to reduce pain and inflammation. A short cold shower, 30 seconds, promotes blood circulation and healing benefits for the entire aching body.

Muscles that are worked consistently and regularly — via a structured work out program to ensure that all the muscles are included — increases in strength. Muscles are made up of elongated muscle cell fibers. These fibers contract, in the power stroke, to produce motion and force. The total force depends on the number and size of these units contracting in unison. Training causes the muscle cells to grow and increase the actin and myosin production, two proteins responsible for contracting the muscles and creating the force of the muscles. Training also causes the muscle fibers to learn to fire in unison, as one, thus increasing maximum power output.

Endurance is the ability of a muscle to continue exerting force without tiring. For endurance, the body is focusing more on the cardiovascular system, ensuring the oxygenated blood reaches all muscles of the body. Two types of muscle fiber — fast-twitch fibers and slow-twitch fibers — are the ones involved when the body is being trained for endurance. Fast-twitch fibers contract quickly but get tired quickly. They use a lot of energy and are useful for sprints. Slow-twitch fibers are best for endurance work; they carry out tasks without getting tired. These are found in core muscles. The type of exercise will promote a type of fiber to be developed. Sprinters have relatively more fast-twitch fibers, as opposed to a long-distance runner, who will have more slow-twitch fibers.

The benefits of exercise are too many to ignore. It is like a magical pill capable of curing a myriad of ills and bring you to your highest level of wellness. There is no excuse for not being engaged in a regular program of exercise. The main reason people do not exercise is lack of interest. If it is not fun, then it is hard to keep doing it. Find some form of exercise that is fun for you. There are tons of different sports and activities one can engage in, either alone or with someone you care about. Make it fun and start a workout program today. An Efenian person is one who exercises regularly, religiously, and they are also very aware of the many benefits of exercising.

Mind Mastery is Thy Tool

The mind is everything. What you think you become

— Buddha

M ind mastery is synonymous with the Buddha. Legend has it that, on the night when Siddhartha Gautama was conceived, Queen Maya had a dream that a white elephant with six white tusks entered her right side and ten months later Siddhartha was born. After Queen Maya became pregnant—according to Shakya tradition—she went to her father's kingdom to give birth. However, her son, Siddhartha—who was to become the Buddha— is said to have been born on the way, at Lumini, what is today Nepal, in a garden beneath a pipal tree.

Siddhartha was born in the 5th century BCE, to a Hindu Kshatriya family. He was the son of Suddhodana, the elected chief of the Shakya Clan. The clan was not a monarchy; it was structured more like an oligarchy. The child was given the name Siddhartha, which means "he who achieves his aim." The prince came into a time where the search for spirituality was common and wide—many major philosophical views were present—people expected spirituality to influence their life in mostly positive ways. Siddhartha grew up in a palace with comforts and luxuries typical of a prince of the times. He was exceptionally intelligent and compassionate. It was predicted that he would become either a great king or a spiritual leader. His parents wanted a great ruler for their kingdom, so they sought to shield the noble prince from the pain and suffering of the world and from the knowledge of human suffering. They surrounded him with all kinds of pleasures. He was given hundreds of the most attractive women to serve his every whim. He was engaged in sports, entertainment, and war training, to prepare him to one day rule the clan. He mastered the art of combat training.

He was raised by his mother's younger sister, Maha Pajapati. Tradition dictated that he was to have the life of a prince. By the time he reached 16, his father had arranged his marriage to a cousin of the same age, Yasodhara, and they fathered a son named Rahula. Siddhartha spent nearly 29 years as a prince in Kapilavastu, while all this time his father provided him with everything one can ever need or want. However, Siddhartha felt empty; all that material wealth he was being provided was not enough to fill his life's ultimate goal. One day, he decided to flee his luxurious palace and venture out into the intriguing city to meet the common people. He is said to have seen an old man. When his charioteer, Chandaka, explained to him that all people grew old, he then decided to go on further trips beyond the palace. On his trip this time, he encountered a diseased man, a decaying corpse, and an ascetic man that inspired him. These events upset him—since this is the first time he had encountered such suffering— as he realized that the world is filled with suffering, sickness, death, and that everyone he loves will at some point go through one of these. The next morning, while the prince was again walking the roads, he walked past a meditator who sat in deep absorption. When he looked at him and their eyes connected, he realized—in a flash of clearness—that the perfection he had been seeking outside must be indeed within one's mind. The meeting with the man gave him a lasting refuge which he knew he had to experience for himself. Siddhartha sought to find a greater meaning to life. Moved by all the things he had experienced, he decided to leave the palace behind, against the will of his father, to live the life of a wandering ascetic. Secretly, in the middle of the night, accompanied by Channa, his servant, and his horse Kanthaka, he left the palace, leaving behind his wife, son, and all the comforts of the prince's life he has been experiencing. He cut his hair, left his horse and servant behind, and journeyed into the woods where he changed into monk's robes. He dedicated himself to meditation and seeking enlightenment amongst the ascetics of the forest. Now living from the sympathy and kindness of others, Siddhartha would beg for food for his sustenance. On one of his begging trips, he went to Rajagaha, where King Bimbisara's men recognized him and the king learned of his quest. King Bimbisara offered him a share of his kingdom, but Siddhartha rejected the offer and told him that his kingdom would be one of the first he would visit after attaining enlightenment.

For six years, he followed the ascetics and fasted to the point that his body wasted away. He would survive for days on a single grain of rice. He met meditation teachers and mastered their techniques. He found that they showed him mind potential but not the mind itself. One day, after many years of wandering in the forest and fasting until the body cried for nourishment, a passing woman gave him some food to eat and afterward he came to the conclusion that torturing the body was not the path to enlightenment. He abandoned the ascetics ways and resolved to follow a "middle path," which was avoiding excesses of both fasting and feasting.

After a journey of many years that would take the future Buddha to experience all life's suffering firsthand, and to study under the master of the times, he decided one day to remain in meditation under a Bodhi tree — fig tree — until the mind's true nature was revealed to him. He was tested every minute while in deep meditation, as his wandering thoughts tried to prevent him from realizing his goal. After a reputed 49 days of meditation, he reached enlightenment on a full moon of May, a week before he turned thirty-five. At the moment of enlightenment, all complexity dissolved and the now Buddha — The Awakened One — experienced the all-encompassing here and now. All separation in time and space disappeared. Past, present, and future all melted into one state of bliss. According to some sutras, at the time of awakening, he realized the complete insight into the Four Noble Truths of the Buddha's principle, thereby attaining liberation from samsara – the endless cycles of birth and rebirth and dying again. Nirvana is the extinguishing of the "fires" of desire, hatred, and ignorance. According to a story in the Samyutta Nikaya, a scripture in the Pali, right after his awakening, the Buddha debated whether he should teach the Dharma to others. He was concerned that humans were so overpowered by ignorance, greed, and hatred that they could never recognize the path, which is subtle, deep, and hard to grasp. In the story of the scriptures, Brahma convinced him to teach, arguing that at least some will understand it. Buddha relented and agreed to teach.

Buddha henceforth decided to spend the rest of his life teaching others how to escape the inherent suffering of life. He traveled for years through India, teaching his philosophy of liberation. His teachings were transmitted primarily orally and not written until many years later after his death. His teachings were of love, compassion, and tolerance. Buddha taught that all living creatures and beings are deserving of compassion. During some of his talks on enlightenment, Buddha would not talk, but just simply held up a flower in his hand and maintained absolute silence. When questioned on this practice later, he would reply that his real teaching could only be understood in silence. Talks could only give limited intellectual information, which was not real enlightenment. He would typically avoid using the word God and, instead, focused on practical ways that a person may escape the cycle of birth and rebirth and attain enlightenment. He spoke in parables and kept his teaching simple and most practical. Buddha encouraged all his followers to question his teaching and to confirm them through their own experiences. Buddha did attract some hostility from jealous competitors. One of his monks, Devadatta, tried to split his community and even tried on three occasions to kill him, but he failed on all attempts. The Buddha passed away after teaching for many years. On his deathbed, he is said to have told his dearest disciple, Ananda, that he should now rely on his teachings and own ethical conduct to be the guide of his life.

The Buddha taught mind mastery through self-inspection, meditation, and a righteous noble way of living. By being virtuous, the Buddha

196

explained one can start the path toward enlightenment. Mind — the collection of conscious and unconscious adaptive mental activities — paired with the body is all of the self. One goes through life growing, adapting, and nurturing one's mind. Mastering the mind entails learning how to be in harmony with oneself — being in control of all of one's emotions and having the fortitude to make rational decisions constantly.

The mind wanders and gets distracted at every moment. One has achieved mastery when this process is purposefully controlled. External and internal stimuli, emotions, and thoughts all conspire to tell the mind how to react. The reptilian brain is primed to jump into action and dictates the reaction needed to keep the body safe; this survival response is a critical function of our brain. However, if we let this reptilian brain take control of all decisions, then mind control is lost, and the interaction is purely animalistic. To be in control, one needs to engage the cerebral cortex part of our brain — the logical brain — and, in a tranquil, grounded manner, makes the logical choice every time: that is mental mastery.

CHAPTER 13: MEET ME AT THE RIVER

MASTERING YOUR MIND

When you become the master of your mind, you are master of everything.

—Swami Satchidananda

What separated us along the evolutionary chain from all other animals was the development of our cerebral cortex. Our big brains, relative to our size, gave us the competitive advantage needed to get to the top of the food chain and basically take over our entire planet. We are 96% genetically similar to our closest relatives, the great ape's species, yet mature apes can barely perform some of the intelligent tasks that a two-year-old human can do. Our brains are the most complex organ in our body. The human brain is as complex as our entire universe. It has an estimated 100 billion neurons, brain cells, each with thousands of connections called synapses which make the brain networks of over one trillion connections. Our brains form a million new connections for every second of our lives. The pattern and strength of the connections are constantly changing, and no two brains are alike. These connections are responsible for storing all our memories. All habits, learning, emotions, personalities, memories, etc., are all etched on our brains in the strength and changing connections of our synapses.

Mind and emotion mastery

Mind mastering refers to being in control of one's actionable thoughts and also having an understanding of how the brain works at a functional, practical, and scientific level. It is by understanding how the brain reacts to what others do to us that we can hope to begin to exercise control of our actions, and not merely react to the environment. One is familiar with the phrase, "*He makes me so mad!*" This is often said as if the stimulus — the person's behavior — causes the reaction (i.e., being mad), without the person having any control of it. When one becomes a master of mind, one starts to take control of this type of situation. Mind mastery refers to controlling your thoughts and your emotions, so you consciously choose your mood and emotional response. If your mind is not used correctly, it can be very detrimental. Your mind (your thoughts) affects your perception of reality. When you change your thoughts, you also change your feelings, as well. By mastering your mind, you control the outcome of emotions and promote a greater level of peace in your mind.

The brain is the Central Processing Unit (CPU) of our body. Philosophers throughout history have believed that the brain may house the essence that makes us human: the soul. The brain is the main organ of the human nervous system; as such, it receives input from all of our senses, and it processes all this information to make sense of its environment. The first records mentioning this organ dated back to Ancient Egyptian medical treatise known as the *Edwin Smith Surgical Papyrus*, named after the man who discovered this document in the seventeenth century. The brain has three main parts. The brainstem connects the brain to the spinal cord and controls the flow of messages between the brain and the rest of the body; it also controls basic body functions such as breathing, swallowing, heart rate, blood pressure, consciousness, and whether one is awake or asleep — referred to as freeze-fight-flight responses. Also, this is our primitive brain. The cerebellum is located at the back of the brain, and it is responsible for regulating movement, motor learning, and maintaining equilibrium. The last part is the cerebrum, the largest part of our brain, and fills up most of the skull; it houses the cerebral cortex and other structures that are responsible for conscious thought, decision-making, memory and learning processes, communication, and perception of external and internal stimuli. The brain is made of soft tissues, which are referred to as gray and white matter (neurons), small blood vessels, and non-neuronal cells which help keep neurons and the rest of the brain's health.

One key question is how we came to have a brain in the first place. Answers to these questions were reviewed by Professor Jon Kass, Vanderbilt University. In his publication, *The evolution of brains from early mammals to humans,* he explains that the early mammals were small, with small brains, an emphasis on olfaction, and little neocortex. Neocortex was transformed from the single layer to six layers of all present-day mammals. Early placental mammals had a corpus callosum connecting the neocortex to the two hemispheres, a primary motor area, and perhaps one or more premotor areas. One line of evolution, he continues, Euarchontoglires, led to present-day primates, tree shrews, flying lemurs, rodents, and rabbits. Early primates evolved from small-brained, nocturnal, insect-eating mammals with an expanded region of the temporal visual cortex. He argues that:

> *Other adaptations included an expansion of the prefrontal cortex and insular cortex. The human and chimpanzee-bonobo lineages diverged some 6–8 million years ago with brains that were about one-third the size of modern humans. Over the last two million years, the brains of our more recent ancestors increased greatly in size, especially in the prefrontal, posterior parietal, lateral temporal, and insular regions. Specialization of the two cerebral hemispheres for related, but different functions became pronounced, and language and other impressive cognitive abilities emerged.*

The oldest part of our brain is an auto-responding section that is responsible for our freeze-flight-fight response, sometimes referred to as the reptilian brain, and it evolved about 500 million years ago. This part of the brain we share with all animals, including reptiles. This reptilian brain is the part of the brain that keeps us alive and away from danger. When danger appears, like a lion on the open savanna, the reptilian drives go on alert. Its system produces a series of hormones that will signal the body to prepare to go on the stress response of freeze-flight-fight. The stress response metabolic parameters raise your heart rate so that more blood is pumped to your legs and muscle in order to be able to run away. The stress response gives priority to all systems needed for the chosen response. Without this alert and response system, the animal will not survive predation or any other life-threatening events. The neocortex, or the thinking part of our brain, is relatively recent when compared to our oldest part. It evolved only about 3 to 4 million years ago. This part of the brain is what makes us uniquely human and give us our key competitive advantage over all other species. The reptilian brain evolved to keep us away from danger but, in today's society, that part of the brain cannot distinguish whether the stress response is coming from trying to escape from a lion or from a rather demanding boss at work. Today, this is one of the main problems, as stress is ever-increasing and, as a result, we have an over-stressed society. The body is in constant stress response which, if sustained for a long time, can have detrimental effects on the body. Chronic disease prevalence is a result of the body being under constant stress response state. Understanding that the stress response is an auto-response, and by being aware of these mechanisms, one can start taking control and making the intelligent response instead of the stress-driven one. In the example above of the demanding boss, an intelligent response would assess the situation and come up with an action plan to address the situation, considering all consequences. This will entail using your cerebral cortex and intelligence, rather than your reactive reptilian brain.

The brain is compartmentalized, and sections of the brain are responsible for different functions. This is not true of higher-order cognitive functions, as different areas of the brain work in concert to create a specific output. The understanding of the inner workings of the brain got a giant leap with the study of the most famous patient in neurology, known as patient HM (Henry G. Molaison). HM was an American memory disorder patient who had a bilateral medial temporal lobectomy to surgically resect the anterior two-thirds of his hippocampi, parahippocampal, entorhinal cortices, piriform cortices, and amygdalae, to cure his epilepsy. The surgery was successful in partially controlling his epilepsy; however, one severe side effect was that he became unable to form new memories. Patient HM was widely studied until his death in 2008. His files were especially important to understanding the theories that explain the link between brain function and memory, and in the development of cognitive neuropsychology. The study revolutionized the current understanding of the organization of human memory. Since patient HM did not have any memory impairment before the surgery, the removal of medial temporal lobes can be held responsible for his memory disorder. This lobe can also be assumed to be a major component involved in the formation of semantic and episodic long-term memories. Despite his amnesic symptoms, HM performed quite normally in the test of intellectual ability, indicating that some memory functions (i.e., short-term, words store, etc.) were not impaired by the surgery. HM was able to remember information over short intervals of time. This finding provides evidence that working memory does not rely on medial temporal structures.

Mind control is the key to understand the world from within us. When we take control of our mind, our ego, our desires, our virtues, and vices are all under the direction of our powerful self—the inner voice that advises us on what is the right thing to do under any circumstances, and with cool and collected, cerebral, cortex-driven thoughts and reasoning. Consider a puppeteer putting up a show on a street filled with bright-eyed, cheerful, and joyful children. He keeps the children fixated on the scene and he awakes the puppets, which seem almost alive under the artful moves of his hands and strings. The puppeteer is controlling the puppets. The hands are moving the puppets; the puppets will never move the hands. It is this one direction that we must understand when dealing with the daily stress and actions of the living world. One sometimes feels like other aspects of one's lives are controlling one. Your job is creating stress, your family is putting too much pressure on you to perform, etc. This is the hand moving the puppets. One is the puppeteer. One makes the decision on how one is going to react to the different stresses that one experiences. If you think of a funny situation that makes you laugh, you say, "It was funny, and I laughed." But it was you that decided to bring about an honest smile. The event seems automatic and without thinking, but one is in control of one's internal action, even actions that are reflex-driven in nature (this will take a higher level of mastery to control). Actors can create smiles on demand and the really good ones are basically indistinguishable from the real smile. When one changes one's thoughts, the body's feelings, a reaction to the world will change. You are in control of mind and emotions. It will need discipline, practice, and knowledge to get to a level of mastery of one's mind.

We know what we are, but know not what we may be.

— William Shakespeare

Mind and emotional mastery return control to thyself. There are seven factors that one must fully understand and apply in one's daily life in order to achieve mind mastery. These are:

1. **Brain knowledge:** One must have a basic understanding of how the brain works, what makes it work, and what makes it ill. There are still a lot of areas of the brain that we do not fully understand yet, but we have come a long way to understand its evolution, functions, and inner-working. Knowledge is power; by understanding the brain's workings, we gain control power back.

2. **Meditation:** Meditation is a way to reboot your brain. It offers a time for the brain to rewire itself and make its connections stronger and healthy. We will explore in a later chapter more in-depth the benefits of meditation to brain functions.

3. **Laughter:** Stress is the main cause of all ills. When we laugh, we practice full relaxation and stress elimination. In a reduced or a low-stress environment, the brain thrives. By practicing humor, we give the brain a chance to de-stress, relax, and grow.

4. **Networking:** We are a connectome, a series of neuron connections that determine who we are. All that is human is encoded in these connections. We should focus on making these connections as strong as possible. To strengthen our connections internally, we should work on our external social connections. Humans are social creatures; we thrive in social environments. When we make our families, our friends, our social connections a priority in our daily lives, we strengthen our internal brain connections. By building positive and productive networks, we record beneficial experiences on our brains.

5. **Empathy:** We are hard-wired for empathy. The brain has "mirror-neurons" which mirror activities we experience. When we are faced with someone in a distressed situation, we "feel" their distress; our mirror-neurons create the situation in us. When we allow the feeling of empathy, when we start to care for more than just ourselves, we have reached a higher level of consciousness. This mature view of our interdependence, our shared humanity, allows us to master our mind by helping put it all in perspective, to start working on our life purpose. Practice, also, kindness and compassion with others as well as oneself. These lead to mind peacefulness and contentment.

6. **Purpose:** Find your life's purpose and plot a course of action to accomplish it. When we find our purpose, we discover our motivation and we can use this fuel to give us the direction we need to follow in our daily affairs. Your personal vision should incorporate your purpose. Create specific goals aligned with your vision.

7. **Emotional Intelligence:** Mastering your mind entails mastering your emotions. Emotions live in the realm of "stress-response." These are important for survival, but when we are emotional, we are engaging our reptilian brain. One should strive to use one's analytical brain as much as possible. No decision of importance should be made when under the influence of the reptilian brain. Emotional intelligence is being aware of the mode you are operating in and act accordingly. If you are in the stress response mode, stop, take a deep breath, assess the situation, and make use of your cerebral cortex to make the decision. Do not worry about things one cannot control; instead, focus on what you can control.

Someone else's actions should not determine your response

— Dalai Lama

Ego is the Latin word for "I." It was popularized by psychologist Sigmund Freud (the founder of psychoanalysis) when he used it as one of three parts to the personality: the ego, the id, and the superego. Psychologists use the term ego in a Freudian sense (i.e., ego, Freud defined as the organized, realistic agent that mediates, between the instinctual desires of the id and the critical super-ego). The general public uses the word ego simply to mean one's sense of self-worth. In this sense, your ego is your conscious mind, the part of your identity that considers your "self". When one says, you have a big ego, one is meaning to say you are full of yourself. A reasonable amount of one own self-worth is a good thing; the key is finding the balance point. The ego is limited and bound; it fears the unknown, and it struggles to get what it wants. The central theme of the ego is insecurity. To take back control, one needs to be able to manage one's ego. A healthy dosage of ego is not only good but necessary. However, when we become egocentric and operate on one of the extremes of the ego scale, then we suffer. One way to manage your ego is to practice self-kindness. When one is kind to oneself, one nourishes and approves oneself, thus finding peace and inner fulfillment without the need to have feelings of jealousy and or frustration of others. Be aware of your ego and where you are at any time on the ego scale, and by so doing, one can start mastering this portion of oneself.

Mastering others is strength. Mastering yourself is true power

— Lao Tzu

Self-sabotage occurs when part of one's personality acts in conflict and interferes with one's long-term goals. Some examples of this type of behavior include drug abuse, comfort eating, procrastination, self-injury, and self-medication. To stop self-sabotage, one must first recognize that one is getting in one's way, then one has a chance to correct the behavior. This self-awareness gets easier as we practice mind and emotion mastery. The body and the mind work as one perfectly harmonized unit. The body is self-healing and self-regulating, so as we become aware of the damaging behavior, the body, with the aid of the mind, can start the healing process.

Do not dwell in the past, do not dream of the future, concentrate the mind on the present moment.

— Buddha

Living in the present —mindfulness

Living in the present is the key to experiencing happiness, because "the here and now, the present" is the only point we have access to; the past is gone, and the future is yet to come. Being present or living in the present means to be mindful of what is happening at the moment, not being distracted by events and or worries in the past or in the future. Being present-minded is the key to holistic health and happiness. It helps with stress reduction, anxiety, worries, and rumination, and keeps you connected to your living environment. Mindfulness is the psychological process of purposely bringing one's attention to experiences occurring in the present moment without judgment. Several clinical studies have proven the benefits of mindfulness to both physical and mental health. The practice of mindfulness seems also to have significant therapeutic benefits to people with psychiatric disorders. Studies also show a reduction in rumination and worries.

Psychologist and author, Ryan M. Niemiec, and his colleagues, have offered an alternative definition of mindfulness. Being mindful, they argued, is not taking things for granted. Mindfulness challenges us to awaken from our mind-habits and appreciate the little things. They expand by their definition by stating that mindfulness means to return to the present moment. No one's mind stays in the present moment. Considering the nature of our mind, it needs to process and compute every moment. We cannot control our mind to chronically stay in the present, but we can have control over the return, we can always return our mind to the present moment. Finally, they stated that mindfulness is the self-regulation of attention with an attitude of curiosity, openness, and acceptance.

Our greatest glory is not in never falling, but in rising every time we fall.

—Confucius

Positivism - a gate to heaven

A positive state of mind refers to choosing favorable outcomes for all life situations. A positive-minded person will consider all possible outcomes but will choose the positive one every time. Traditional folklore refers to looking at a glass has full, rather than half empty. Psychologists called it positive psychology. They define positive psychology as the study of the "good life", or the positive aspects of the human experience. This focus is not only on the individual but also on society as well. Consider your daily mind state. Are you positive most of the time? Are you pessimistic?

Positivism eliminates negativism and improves living. It can be used as a tool to increase happiness and self-actualization. Studies have shown that optimists have a better life than pessimists. A study from Harvard T.H. Chan School of Public Health[53] found that having an optimistic outlook on life, a general expectation that good things will happen, may help people live longer. The study found that optimistic women have a significantly reduced risk of dying from several major causes of death, including cancer, heart disease, stroke, respiratory disease, and infection. The study commented: "Our new findings suggest that we should make efforts to boost optimism, which has been shown to be associated with healthier behaviors and healthier ways of coping with life challenges." On the therapy of interventions by increasing optimism, they added that: "Encouraging use of these interventions could be an innovative way to enhance health in the future."

Your thoughts becomes reality; what you thinks about, you brings about. Positive thinking has very real psychological changes in the body resulting in positive outcomes for the body in general. Over 50% of all stress is mental. One approach is to look at life in a positive way to dramatically reduce mental stress. We have a lot of control over this mental stress, by changing our way of thinking and adopting a positive outlook. Happy people have been found to have a stronger immune system and, additionally, they live longer. One can think of one's mood as a self-fulling process: when one embarks on positive thinking then more positive things seem to happen. It also works with negative thoughts, as more negative events will surround you. Given those two choices, it is clear that it is always better to be a positron (a positive and optimistic individual). What one thinks about, comes about. It is said that one's strong thoughts are manifested as if by magic. Sometimes we think we are going to get bad news and, as it happens, bad news appears. The same is true for positive thoughts: if one thinks truly about cash, somehow it magically appears. We call it a self-fulfilling prophecy, or could be the placebo effect. By changing our outlook, we change how we behave around people; the air of confidence produces a reason for others to increase the chances of getting our desired outcome. If you have never experienced this, go ahead and try it—you will be amazed at the results. Why, then, do not people do this all the time? Unfortunately, most people are hardwired for negativity and, after all, the media that one is exposed to every second is only about the negative, tragic, and sensationalized news (they need to sell a product, after all, and they know people are more drawn towards negative and dramatic news). When was the last time you heard on the news report of a fellow citizen helping a homeless person to get back on their feet, or of someone assisting an old lady with her groceries? This feel-good act of kindness is not worthy of news time, according to our current media business. The mind and body are internally connected. Your thoughts, your perceptions of the world are what really matters. Reality is of minor importance; It is what you think of the event that matters or, in order words, how your particular brain is reading the given situation. Interpretation of any event is a function of the particular brain in question. Two individuals can both experience the same event. For one, the event could be so dramatic that he would consider suicide, while, for the other person, the same event may just be a minor distraction. It is not that event that matters, but how you view and perceive it. One needs to constantly retrain one's brain to access one's reality as the most positive one. This, in turn, will maximize our happiness.

CHAPTER 14: A KITE IN THE WIND

MEDITATION — THE ART OF BREATHING

To a mind that is still. The whole universe surrenders.

—Anonymous

M editation dates back thousands of years and it is a practice that has been used by monks, Buddhists, and other religious traditions to obtain enlightenment and self-realization. It is primarily a technique where one uses mindfulness, mental focus, or other tools to train attention and awareness to achieve mental clarity and an emotionally calm and stable state. Some of the earliest written records of meditation come from the Hindu traditions of Vedantism. The word meditation is derived from Latin *meditatio,* meaning "to think, contemplate, devise, ponder." The nattering, chattering voices in our head seem never to leave us alone. Meditation gives one the means to quiet the mind, to stop the chatter that keeps increasing our stress levels and preventing us from sleeping. Additionally, by helping us clear our minds and eliminate brain fog, meditation promotes self-fulfillment and enlightenment. Several studies have documented the many benefits of meditations and these include improvement of the immune system, less anxiety, less depression, reduced stress levels, increasing peace and perception, a heightened sense of well-being, fulfillment, and overall greater happiness.

Meditation—mind exercise and healing

Hundreds of studies have been conducted on the effect of meditation on the human brain. Modern scientific techniques, such as fMRI, EEG, have been used to observe neurological responses during meditation. Psychologists have developed mindfulness practice meditation to alleviate mental and physical conditions. It has also been used to treat drug addiction, depression, stress, and anxiety. A meta-analysis study was done in 2017 on the effects of meditation on empathy, compassion, and prosocial behaviors; it found that meditation practices have small to medium effects on self-reported and observable outcomes, concluding that such practices can improve positive prosocial emotions and behaviors.

Meditation history can be attributed to early religions. Buddhist scholar B. Alan Wallace mentioned that focused attention is a basis for the practice of mindfulness. He said, "Truly effective meditation is impossible without focused attention." Matt Rossano argues that the emergence of the capacity for focused attention, a key element of meditation, may have contributed to the latest phases of human biological evolution. He writes, "Campfire rituals of focused attention created Baldwinian selection for enhanced working memory among our Homo sapiens ancestors. This emergence was in part caused by a fortuitous genetic mutation that enhanced working memory capacity". In the 5th century BCE, other forms of meditation appeared: Confucianism and Taoism in China, Hinduism, Jainism, and Buddhism in India. By the

20 BCE, the Roman Empire had written on some form of spiritual exercises involving attention and concentration and, by the 3rd century, Plotinus developed meditative techniques. The Silk Road transmission of Buddhism introduced meditation to several Asian countries and, by 653, the first meditation hall was opened in Singapore.

There are several classifications of meditation but, in the West, two have dominated: focused (or concentrative) meditation and open (or mindfulness) meditation. The focused attention meditation refers to focusing attention on an object, breathing, image, or words (mantra). Transcendental meditation is this type of meditation. Open meditation includes mindfulness and other awareness states. The benefits of meditation extend to all types of meditation. The positive effects on the body and mind arise from the fact that meditation allows the brain time to reboot. When one practices calming the mind and breathing properly, one gives the body and mind the fuel required to elevate both to the highest level of performance.

The benefits of medication have been confirmed by hundreds of studies. The key benefits include:

1. **Lower stress:** A study published on the US National Library of Medicine found that mindful meditation showed reduced anxiety, less depression, less pain, and, to a small level, also improvement of mental health-related quality of life. This study included 3,515 participants and randomized clinical trials, accounting for placebo effects and sufficient statistical confidence level. There is a lot of evidence correlating stress with illness: the higher the stress level, the higher the levels of illness. Meditation helps decrease stress. Mental, physical, and chemical stressors can be traced back to the cause of every illness. When the body is under stress, it releases cortisol. In the short term, this is a beneficial response, but the issue arises when one is under long term stress and the body is constantly producing this hormone. Long term cortisol has many harmful effects, such as chronic inflammation. The

stress level can disrupt sleep, promote depression and anxiety, increase blood pressure, fatigue, and cloudy thinking. In an eight-week study, mindfulness meditation was found to reduce the inflammation response caused by the stress. Research also has demonstrated that meditation may improve symptoms of stress-related conditions like irritable bowel syndrome, post-traumatic stress disorder, and fibromyalgia.

2. **Improve focus and memory function**: Meditation has been shown to improve focus and memory functions. One difference I noticed when I started meditating regularly was how easy it was to recall facts and memories, and I noticed a heightened ability to focus intently and longer. A review of twelve studies found that meditation increased attention, memory, and quickness in older volunteers. Meditation can not only help the age-related memory loss but also it has been found to partially improve memory in patients with dementia. By improving focus and memory, one is helping the brain stay young, sharp, and optimally fine-tuned. The additional focus gained through meditation contributes to mental clarity and better memory. Another review on meditation found that meditation may even reverse patterns in the brain that contribute to mind-wandering, worrying, and poor attention. One can reap the benefits of these meditation practices even with practice as short as four times a week. The key is to get started practicing meditation and keep improving the techniques.

3. **Control anxiety:** The American Psychological Association (APA) defines anxiety as an emotion characterized by a feeling of tension, worried thoughts, and physical changes like increased blood pressure. People with anxiety disorders usually have intrusive thoughts or concerns. They may also show physical symptoms such as sweating, trembling, dizziness, or rapid heartbeat. Meditation acts to

reduce stress, thereby reducing anxiety. A study followed eighteen volunteers three years after they had completed an eight-week meditation program. Most of them have been continuing with their meditation practice and they were found to have lower levels of anxiety over the long term, Meditation was also found to reduce symptoms associated with anxiety disorders, such as phobias, social anxiety, paranoid thoughts, obsessive-compulsive behavior, and panic attacks. Job-related anxiety due to a high-pressure work environment has also been found to be attenuated and eliminated in some cases. One study found meditation reduced anxiety in a group of nurses.

4. **Decrease depression:** Per APA, "depression is more than just sadness, they add that people with depression may experience a lack of interest and pleasure in daily activities, significant weight loss or gain, insomnia or excessive sleeping, lack of energy, inability to concentrate, feelings of worthlessness or excessive guilt and recurrent thoughts of death or suicide". Depression is one of the most common mental disorders; fortunately, it is very treatable. Research has found that some form of meditation can improve depression and, in general, create a positive outlook on life. Two studies on mindful meditation found decreased depression in over 4,600 adults. Several studies suggest that meditation may reduce depression by decreasing body inflammatory chemicals, called cytokines. Other mechanisms suggested by other studies claim that electrical activity in those who practiced mindfulness meditation shows measurable changes in activity levels in areas related to positive thinking and optimism.

5. **Improve self-awareness:** Being self-aware refers to being able to recognize how others and how one's own feelings are affecting the self. Meditation may help one develop a stronger understanding of oneself, thus helping one grow and be the best one can be. At times, one can be self-

sabotaging and one's negative thoughts can be self-defeating and lead to harm of oneself and or others. Self-inquiry meditation aims to help one develop a better understanding of one's self. By starting to know oneself better, one's tendencies, thoughts and emotions, and reactions to a stimulus, one can start making positive changes.

6. **Improve sleeping:** Sleeping disorders are quite common in our modern society. We have a sleep-deprived society and most people are not getting enough sleep to keep their body functioning at their optimum. The American Sleep Association (ASA) reports that 50 to 70 million US adults have a sleep disorder. Drowsy driving accounts for 1,550 fatalities and 40,000 nonfatal injuries annually in the United States. 37.9% report unintentionally falling asleep during the day at least once in the preceding month. Meditation has been found to help one fall asleep faster and stay asleep longer than those who do not meditate. Meditation techniques can help one to relax better, to control the mind, and avoid those troubling thoughts that prevent us from sleeping. This not only reduces the time it takes to fall asleep but also improves the quality of sleep.

7. **Promotes love and kindness:** Metta meditation, a type of meditation also known as loving-kindness meditation, may increase positive feelings and actions toward oneself and others. This meditation begins with the self and gradually extends the wish for well-being happiness to all beings. By practicing this type of meditation, one learns to extend kindness and forgiveness externally, first to friends, then to acquaintances, and ultimately to enemies. Twenty-two studies on this form of meditation have shown its ability to increase people's compassion toward themselves and others. Another study showed the positive feelings developed through Metta meditation can improve social

anxiety, help anger management, and even reduce marriage conflicts. Also, the effect seems to be cumulative; that is, the more one is exposed to this type of meditation, the more positive feeling one experiences.

Daily meditation—mindful awareness

With the laundry list of benefits, one gets from meditation, it is very puzzling why not everyone is doing it. The answer is a combination of culture, lack of knowledge of these techniques, and overall excuses involving the amount of time required to meditate. Meditation is something everyone can do and should do to improve mental and emotional health. It can be done just about anywhere, with no special equipment or places needed.

There are many types of meditation, but regardless of which type and even if one only practice for a few minutes, one will benefit and improve the quality of life. Choose a meditation style that best suits you and start practicing. Here are some simple steps to start. One should start with 5 minutes a day and gradually increase it to about 20 minutes twice a day.

- *Find a quiet place* in your house (bathrooms are ideal places), sit in a comfortable position with feet on the ground and hands in your lap, and hands facing toward the ceiling. Once one gets more advanced, a yoga position would be best.
- *Close your eyes* and focus your thought on your breathing. Relax your body. As thoughts come in, just let them go by; eventually, they will fade away altogether.
- One can *use a mantra* (like Aum). Repeat your mantra rhythmically and in harmony with your breath. Make your breath full, slowly inhaling and exhaling from deep inside. One's goal is to completely let go. Set an alarm but do not be tempted to look at it. Just focus on your breathing, mantra, and staying totally relaxed.

- If you recognize a thought, *simply keep up with your mantra and breathing*, and it will float away.
- After your time is up, *open your eyes*, sit for a few minutes more until you feel ready to continue with your day.

The key to meditation is to get started. The very first time you start, do not be concerned with having a mind clear of thoughts. Meditation mastering takes decades, if not longer, to get good at; one's main concern when starting is on consistency and persistence. One should keep at it until it feels natural and comfortable. If one practices meditation daily, one will get to the point where the practice is one of enjoyment, and one would be looking forward to the time to meditate.

Oxygen—cell vitality

Oxygen is the lifeblood of every cell, and we get it when we breathe the air around us. Oxygen is very important to live and, in fact, life as we know it cannot exist without it. Although breathing is as natural as living, most people do not know how to breathe properly. Breathing is one of the key techniques in most martial arts to control the strength of the body and find body and mind balance. Whenever you encounter a stressful situation, breathe deep and fully for fifteen seconds and you will notice your stress starts melting away. Proper and deep oxygenation revitalizes all your cells and promotes overall body functioning. Oxygen is a vital component of every single cell in your body. All forms of life are made of cells and each one requires energy. Oxygen fuels the cells and provides the basic building blocks they need to survive. The cells combine oxygen with nitrogen and hydrogen to produce several proteins that, in turn, build new cells. Daily, about seven hundred billion cells in our bodies wear out and must be replaced; oxygen helps build these new cells.

Respiration, and the absorption of oxygen, help convert the nutrients we eat to fuel the cells needed to thrive. Oxygen is also important to our immune system. It is used to help kill bacteria by fueling the cells that make up our body's defenses. The process used by the body to convert food into energy is the process of combustion. This process is slow rate combustion taking place in the mitochondria of the cell. Mitochondria — sometimes refers to as the powerhouse of the cell — are specialized organelles within the cell. They use specialized enzymes to transfer the energy released from the oxidation of our food to a storage molecule called adenosine triphosphate (ATP). ATP is the currency of the body; it delivers energy within the cells of the body, thus maintaining the chemical reactions needed for the cells to function normally. Respiration occurs within the cell and the nutrient fuel is burned with oxygen to release energy. The respiratory system, the nose, trachea, lungs, circulatory system, and related muscles, all act to transport oxygen from the air we breathe and bring it to every individual cell of the body. If any of these organs is not functioning properly or any of them is altered in any way, energy production would be changed as well. If follows, then, that when one does not get enough oxygen to meet the body's energy needs, then the cells do not get the energy they need to function properly. This leads to cell atrophy and sometimes even death.

Health is causally related to the quality of our breathing. Depending on our current state, joy, fear, anger, etc., we experience changes in the breathing patterns. The breathing can be diaphragmatic, continuous, interrupted, rhythmic, or irregular. If we intentionally or unconsciously change our breathing patterns, it will affect our physical and emotional state. To correct the ill effect of improper breathing patterns, one needs to pay attention to how air is coming in and out of the body, practicing quality breathing. Correct breathing means breathing in a physiologically optimal way that the body was designed for. Some common bad breathing habits include, for example, over-breathing, chest breathing, and holding your breath. These bad habits lead to a shortage of oxygen, of energy, and they end up stressing the body. To solve these bad habits, it is imperative one is aware of one's breathing habits and then one consciously and purposely turns them into the correct ones.

Bad breathing patterns lead to several adverse effects on the body. Improper breathing creates tension on the body which increases the stress on the body. The airways also get tighter as a result of bad breathing forcing the body to work harder and breathe faster. Blood vessels could also constrict, which leads to higher blood pressure and increases the load on the heart. Additionally, bad breathing decreases the body's ability to deliver oxygen to the cells, resulting in reduced cell development and growth. Organs of the body also get affected negatively when one's breath is inadequate. The brain uses twenty percent of the oxygen we consume. If the brain lacks oxygen, then lots of its functions would be affected as well. Lack of oxygen to the heart means it cannot pump blood as efficiently as it is able, which leads to bad circulation and heart issues. Muscles get affected, as well, by lack of proper oxygenation, which can result in lower physical performance.

Nature, through the process of evolution, has provided Homo sapiens with an extremely efficient respiratory system. To breathe correctly, we should follow the naturally defined process of respiration. The nose is perfectly adapted for airflow. One should start by breathing in and out through the nose. The nose is equipped with an optimal air cleaning system consisting of hair, mucous membranes, and channels designed to keep away pathogens and to prepare the air to enter the body. When one breathes through the mouth, one is bypassing this perfectly adapted air purifying system. Additionally, mouth breathing provides the lungs with unfiltered air, which is full of viruses and bacteria that may not be beneficial to the body. It may take some time to get used to breathing through your nose, but if one continues practicing nose breathing, the body gets used to it. It could take a few days to get fully used to breathing this way.

Diaphragm breathing promotes deep and full breaths. The air you breathe should be deep enough that you should feel the chest rising rhythmically every time one takes a breath. 70-80 percent of the inhaling should be done by the diaphragm. Diaphragm breathing helps circulate much of the air in the lower parts of the lungs. It also helps the lymphatic system get rid of waste products. The rhythmic motion of diaphragm breathing makes the chest, shoulder, and neck more relaxed, reducing or eliminating pains in these areas. Additionally, it decreases the pressure in the chest and belly, resulting in a heart that does not have to work as hard.

Relaxed breathing refers to being in a state of relaxation while breathing. One can take advantage of the periodicity of the breathing motion to promote relaxation. Be aware of any tension on the body and get rid of it. The up and down patterns of relaxed breathing create calmness, stress reduction, and an optimally functioning body. Bodies in the lowest stress level are the highest functioning ones. Harmonious breathing means taking rhythmic and quiet breaths that are in tune with one natural frequency. Think of waves in a calm ocean and try to mimic the frequency of the wave in one's breathing pattern. Being in an upright, erect position helps promote harmonious breathing as well. When we speak, we breathe louder; this leads to incorrect breathing. Being aware of one's pattern is a sure way to correct bad breathing. One should frequently monitor breathing patterns and act accordingly. By practicing daily and taking corrective actions, one can revert to proper breathing once more.

PART SEVEN: THE SEVENTH NOBLE TRUTH

Networks are Thyself

LOOK AGAIN AT THAT DOT. THAT'S HERE. THAT'S HOME. THAT'S US. ON IT EVERYONE YOU LOVE, EVERYONE YOU KNOW, EVERYONE YOU EVER HEARD OF, EVERY HUMAN BEING WHO EVER WAS, LIVED OUT THEIR LIVES. THE AGGREGATE OF OUR JOY AND SUFFERING, THOUSANDS OF CONFIDENT RELIGIONS, IDEOLOGIES, AND ECONOMIC DOCTRINES, EVERY HUNTER AND FORAGER, EVERY HERO AND COWARD, EVERY CREATOR AND DESTROYER OF CIVILIZATION, EVERY KING AND PEASANT, EVERY YOUNG COUPLE IN LOVE, EVERY MOTHER AND FATHER, HOPEFUL CHILD, INVENTOR, AND EXPLORER, EVERY TEACHER OF MORALS, EVERY CORRUPT POLITICIAN, EVERY "SUPERSTAR," EVERY "SUPREME LEADER," EVERY SAINT AND SINNER IN THE HISTORY OF OUR SPECIES LIVED THERE—ON A MOTE OF DUST SUSPENDED IN A SUNBEAM.

—CARL SAGAN

Networks can be simply defined as a group formed from parts that are connected. As Homo sapiens, we are a large group, connected by our shared humanity. We are a network! Networks are abundant in our lives and they play a key role in our everyday routines. As social creatures, we crave networks that allow us to stay connected to our fellow humans, to share ideas, communicate feelings, and express our emotions. The need to share with others is basic to our existence. Productive and effective social networks, friend networks, family networks, and professional networks all must be maintained and nurtured in order to achieve a balanced life and happiness. Without these, one would feel lonely, lack purpose, and have a strong sense of not belonging. Positive social networks feed our soul and nurture the spirit.

The brain, the most complex organ in the universe, is a finely tuned network system. It contains over eighty billion neurons, and each is connected to about ten thousand other neurons forming the neural network, like branches on a tree, this is what we call a neural network. The neural network defines us and provides us with consciousness and that characteristic we call humanity. We are a network in the biological and social sense of the word.

Carl Sagan, a prominent astronomer, cosmologist, astrophysicist, author, and science communicator, is the ambassador of our shared humanity, our connected nature as human beings. He argued for our similarity as human beings, for sharing our common home – earth – and for ensuring that we are all guardians of our earth and of each other. He showed us through his communications and books that the universe is vast, and we are just a small speck of dust in its immensity. By being humble, respectful of all life on our planet and beyond, and by treating each other ethically, we can create networks of connections worthy of our humanity.

He was a very well-known scientist during the decades of the '70s and '80s. He hosted the famous TV show, "Cosmos: A Personal Voyage". He studied extraterrestrial intelligence, advocated for nuclear disarmament, wrote several books and academic papers. Carl was born in 1934, in Brooklyn, New York to a Russian immigrant family. His father, Samuel Sagan, was a garment worker and his mother, Rachel Molly Gruber, was a housewife. He also had a sister, Carol, and all lived in a small apartment in Bensonhurst, in Brooklyn. According to Carl, they were Reform Jews – the most liberal kind of Judaism. Carl would say that his father was not religious; however, his mother "definitely believed in God, and was active in the temple ... and served only *kosher* meat."

Carl, the first of two children, began his interest in astronomy very early in his life. At the early age of five, his mother would send the curious Carl to the library to find books on stars. His parents, to nurture his interest in astronomy — when he was four years old — took him to the 1939 New York World's Fair, where visions of the future inspired him and further fueled his interest in the cosmos and the future. The show displayed photoelectric cells which created a crackling sound, while other exhibits showed little General Motors cars carrying people to skyscrapers, all combining to spark his interest in futuristic technology and speculations. He thereafter became a fan of the science-fiction stories in pulp magazines, and of the flying saucers and extraterrestrial life depicted in these narratives. Carl would claim that his sense of wonder came from his father, who in his free time gave apples to the poor and worked to ease tension between labor and management in the garment industry. In his later writing, he would describe his parent's influence: "My parents were not scientists. They knew almost nothing about science. But in introducing me simultaneously to skepticism and to wonder, they taught me the two uneasily cohabiting modes of thought that are central to the scientific method."

After graduating from high school in 1951, Carl went to the University of Chicago to pursue his degree and work on his interests in the possibility of alien life. This was one of few schools that would consider admitting a 16-years-old student. The school was ideal for him in the sense that it had some of the nation's leading scientists — Enrico Fermi and Edward Teller — working there, operating the famous Yerkes Observatory. In 1960, he earned his Ph.D. with a thesis on *Physical Studies of Planets*. During the '60s, he worked at Harvard University and the Smithsonian Astrophysical Observatory, focusing on the physical conditions of the planets. In 1968, he became director of Cornell University's Laboratory for Planetary Studies, and three years later become a full professor. He also worked with NASA — National Aeronautics and Space Administration — to help them choose where the Viking probes would explore Mars; he also helped NASA craft the messages that were sent with the Pioneer and Voyager probes set to go beyond our solar system.

He was one of the most famous scientist of his time, due in part to the books he wrote: *The Cosmic Connection: An Extraterrestrial Perspective (1973), Other Worlds (1975), The Dragons of Eden: Speculations on the Evolution of Human Intelligence (1977*; Pulitzer Prize winner) and his 1985 novel, *Contact*. His novel, *Contact*, was made into a popular science fiction movie starring Judie Foster. By 1980, he had co-founded the Planetary Society—an international nonprofit organization focusing on space exploration. During this time, he was also the host of the very influential TV series, "Cosmos: A Personal Voyage", which went on to educate and inspire thousands of future engineers and scientists. One of his most famous works, *Pale Blue Dot: A Vision of the Human Future in Space* (1994) was inspired by the famous Pale Blue Dot picture, which shows Earth as a mere speck in space. Carl convinced NASA to turn Voyager 1 one last time as it exited the solar system and to take a picture of our planet, the last home picture, as it went into the abyss of open space to forever evidence our existence. Voyager 1 was about four billion miles away when it captured its final portrait of our world. Caught in the center of scattered light rays, the earth appears as a tiny point of light, a point he called a pale blue dot. Carl was honored several times during his notable career, receiving NASA's Distinguished Public Service Medal (1977, 1981) and the National Academy of Sciences Public Welfare medal (1994), just to mention a few. Carl died of pneumonia from a complication of the bone-marrow disease myelodysplasia, at the age of 62.

By focusing on space, on the outer planets and stars, and on the cosmos, Carl forced us all to look inside each and every one of us, to see ourselves as we are—connected community, with a common home—a shared-humanity. Carl Sagan brilliantly described our shared humanity. We are all embedded on this planet, the place we call home. When one realizes the immensity of space, and how tiny we are in comparison, our daily concern appears minuscule in comparison. Then we realize how important it is to focus on what unites us, not on what divides us. When our shared humanity is recognized, deep connections can be forged across wide cultural divides, which can support both inner and outer peace.

> *Our species needs, and deserves, a citizenry with minds*
> *wide awake and a basic understanding of how the world works*
>
> —Carl Sagan

CHAPTER 15: A SPIDER WEB

NETWORKS—INFORMATION HIGHWAYS

It really boils down to this: that all life is interrelated. We are all caught in an inescapable network of mutuality, tied into a single garment of destiny. Whatever affects one destiny, affects all indirectly.

—Martin Luther King Jr.

Life is a system of networks. The neuro-network is responsible for defining the self. All we are, our memories, emotions, actions, and reactions are imprinted on our connectome (neuro-network). Similar to the neuro-network is our social network. We are social creatures and, as such, we need to be connected to other humans. These networks of support form the basis of our social networks (family networks, friends' networks, work networks, and social networks). By being active participants and by cultivating these networks, we can achieve our highest level of happiness. Studies have shown that loneliness has been related to a wide range of health problems including high blood pressure, cardiovascular diseases, cognitive decline, and immune system deficiencies.

Humans are social creatures. We have evolved to be social creatures as this presents several advantages over the alternative: lonely, single existence. Our early ancestors realized what group living can offer them: improved predator detection, improved resource detection, an opportunity for cooperation, reduced risk of infanticide, and increased opportunity for social learning. With this communal living comes some negative consequences, as well: pathogen transmission (due to close proximities), resource allocation (sharing), competition, aggression, and cognitive capabilities, as more information must be analyzed. However, the benefits far outweigh the disadvantages and that is why today we continue to look for more and more ways to connect to one another.

Healing yourself is connected with healing others.

——Yoko Ono

Support networks—mental relaxation

When asked if they have someone they can go to for support, many Americans answer that they do not feel they have enough support. According to experts, more than 55 percent said they could use a little more social support. It is a fact that most people can benefit from social and emotional support. Having a strong support network can make one more able to cope with problematic situations and can improve self-esteem. However, building this support network requires some work and diligence; it does not happen naturally or automatically; one needs to purposely build this network. This network consists of your social support, your family, your friends, your colleagues, and your social environments; all are part of your circle of happiness networks. When this network is well built and strong, it increases our wellbeing. Focusing on nurturing this network should be one of our key priorities.

One does not need an exceptionally large network to realize the benefits of networking. A practical, symbiotic group of friends and family will produce just as much benefit as a large network. When considering your networks of support, look to the people you interact with, as this will be a natural way to grow your network. Most networks are made of feedback loops; that is to say, that the communication is not just one way but is circular in nature. If one is only concerned with getting benefits and advantages from the relationship and not sharing or giving back (i.e., the feedback loop), the system will break down. If you are there for others, they will be there for you when the need arises. Some research has shown that providing social support is more important than receiving it. An honest relationship of all parties involved is one that is concerned with the wellbeing of the group, not just a single individual. The members of your network of support should be people that you can trust, people who are reliable and positive-thinking individuals. You have to be very proactive to build all your networks; it takes dedication to create powerful and productive networks, but once done, it is worthwhile.

To be effective at networking one needs to learn and practice social skills. Look to enjoy the experience as one gets to know others. Consider joining groups that have similar interests to yours. Nowadays, with the advent of the internet, there are thousands of different groups one can interact with and get to know better. Consider also traditional meeting places as sources of relationships, like your religious organizations, charities, national organizations, community centers, etc.

Grow and feed your brain networks. With connections being created in your brain every time we have new experiences; we have a myriad of opportunities to grow the neural network. One can create positive memories, with beneficial future potential, or negative ones; you choose. It is your interpretation of the world that creates your internal model of reality. Based on this, one should focus on a positive outlook and experiences to create neuronal connections that help us, not hurt us. Create body-mind connections that promote mental and physical health. One can think of "possibility for action" when having to make a choice of the type of experiences to create and nurture. Imagine someone asks you, "What do you think of my new outfit? One can be honest and tell that

228

person what is really in one's mind and the truth of what one thinks of the crazy clothes they are wearing. However, if one thinks of the possibilities for the action of such an answer, then the answer becomes crystal clear. What possibility for action will I get with the response that I am about to give? Is it worth it to pursue this course of thinking? Will it be a positive response? By applying these tools, one will come up with the right answer every time. Next time you are faced with a difficult dilemma, think, "What is the possibility for action of my response?"

There are several things to keep in mind when developing fruitful networks of support, whether it is networks of friendships, family, profession, or pure social networks. Is the relationship a trustworthy one? One should base the relationship on trust with each other, and the communication should be open, honest, and of mutual respect. Also consider diversity when creating your networks. Diversity is the mechanism that natural selection uses to optimize the species; we can use diversity, as well, to create better networks. Diversity offers different points of view, which are the genesis of ideas and creative thinking.

Our shared humanity binds us together

Horrible things can happen when our focus lies on our differences rather than our similarities. In 1994, members of the Hutu ethnic majority in Rwanda brutally slaughtered as many as 800,000 people, mostly Tutsi minorities (seventy-five percent of the Tutsi population). Hutu nationalists in the capital of Kigali spread the genocide through the country with shocking speed and brutality, as neighbors killed neighbors, families turned on families, love turned to hate, and ordinary citizens everywhere were incited by local officials and the Hutu government to take up arms. All these people were killed in a period of fewer than 100 days. By the time, the Tutsi-led Rwandese Patriotic Front gained control of the country through a military offensive, hundreds of thousands of Rwandans laid dead, and more than 2 million refugees had fled Rwanda. Genocide, considered the worst crime against humanity, is the planned mass killing of a racial, ethnic, or religious group. Based on this definition, the Rwanda genocide was one of the worst in history, and the rate of killing (six men, women, and children slaughtered every minute of every day for 100 days), was five times higher than that of the holocaust of World War II. Hutu gangs searched out victims hiding in Churches and school buildings. The militia murdered victims with machetes and rifles. The Hutu gangs recruited and pressured civilians to arm themselves with machetes, clubs, blunt objects, and other weapons, and encouraged them to rape, maim, and kill their Tutsi neighbors, and to destroy or steal their property. The goal was to kill every Tutsi living in Rwanda. Rape was used as a weapon. The genocidaires forced others to stand by during rapes. A testimonial by a woman recalled seeing local people, other generals, and Hutu men watching her get raped about five times a day. What would compel people to do such a heinous crime against people of the same racial origin and of very similar phenotypes and culture? When one focuses on what makes one different, rather than our shared humanity, one can justify unspeakable crimes. These two tribes have so much in common, but there were a few differences. One tribe was more focused on agriculture, while the other was focused on animal farming. Also, they have different migration patterns and social status. These small differences were enough to create an illusion of fear, misinformation, propaganda, and finally brainwashing, to move a herd of people into committing genocide. By focusing on our similarities, rather than our differences one brings out the best in humanity.

CONCLUSION: LIMITLESS LIFE LIVING

ONE NEW DAY—A NEW ME

Wise men talk because they have something to say; fools,
because they have to say something.

—Plato

Y our next chapter in life is yet to be written. Now you have new ink;
henceforward, you shall write your legacy masterpiece, the best
version of you. Our journey into life's most important pursuits—
happiness, a life worth living, and living in the present—have opened a
world of possibilities. We have learned about the seven noble truths and
their applications to all the aspects of life. Now it is your turn to put these
into action. By following through with one's journaling, the unwavering
execution, and one's commitment to the Efenian's way of life, one will
reach the life's highest potential. The recipe to accomplish this is the
Efenian's commitments. I use this term to express the collection of values
that we have reviewed so far. I summarize below all the commitments
that one will need to become an Efenian. Commit to these and you will
be on your way to achieving your highest potential, and to your greatest
level of happiness and fulfillment. To continue to learn and grow on these

231

topics, feel free to review my collection of scientific papers and scientific-based books in the reference section. Remember that one key tool of the Efenian's way of life is being a life-long learner. As such, you will continue the learning journey until the end of your physical existence. Use the noble truths to come up with your own set of unique, customized tools. I've provided several examples of tools you can use to achieve self-fulfillment, but the canvas is only limited by your imagination. The goal is to achieve mastery of the noble truths and then tools to deal with every challenge will be easy to find. Appendix A provides you with a seven-week plan to start your journey. Remember, you are now a life-long learner, an Efenian.

Welcome aboard!

Efenian's Commitments

Internalize, memorize, and apply ALL 7 noble truths!

1st NOBLE TRUTH: The Body is Thy temple

I pledge to treat my body like the "temple" of my soul, to revere it.
I pledge to holistic fitness for life (FQ factor of 90 or better), optimize fitness.

2nd NOBLE TRUTH: Stress-free is Thy Answer

I pledge to eliminate all stresses (chemical, physical and mental) out of my life.

I pledge to love myself, laugh often, and remember that I am unique, powerful, and intelligent.

3rd NOBLE TRUTH: Execution begets Peak Performance

I pledge to execute my actions, be virtuous, and respect all life. All life has equal value.

4th NOBLE TRUTH: Food is Thy Medicine

I pledge to only eat food that heals and grows my body, organic plant-based nutrition.

5th NOBLE TRUTH: Body in Motion is Thy Path

I pledge to frequently exercise and or do physical activity at least 4 times a week.

6th NOBLE TRUTH: Mind Mastery is Thy Tool

I pledge to stay positive and "centered" under any, if not all, situations.

I pledge to be a curious "life-long" learner of all scientific knowledge—cultivate wisdom.

7th NOBLE TRUTH: Networks are Thyself

I pledge to be thankful, generous, and serve others to better humanity.

You may say I am a dreamer, but I am not the only one. I hope

someday you will join us. And the world will live as one

—John Lennon

Efenian—A new road

Now that we have put it all together, we have learned and internalized the seven noble truths and their application to real-life and happiness, we must apply it to our lifestyle, our way of life. To be an Efenian, one must follow the Efenian's commitment and live every day the primal truth of "being the very best version of oneself, one can be an Efenian!":

- Live in the present, every time, every day.
- Be a life-long learner. Knowledge and wisdom are the tools to help understand the world and yourself.
- Smile—frequently, often, and with honest intentions.
- Live life with purpose, find your purpose, create your vision, live it now, today.
- Be a positron: positive people live longer and more satisfying lives.
- Be in control of your mind and emotions. You are the master of your destiny.
- Be generous and kind. Practice random acts of kindness.
- Time heals what reason cannot. Be aware that time is finite. Use every second wisely.
- Master the seven noble truths and one can generate one's own tools of productivity and happiness.

Share these values with the people you love, and the world would be a much more pleasant place to live.

Appendix A: My Seven-Week Plan

My seven-week plan

This is a seven-week plan to become the best version of you. Follow these steps and get started on the journey of your life. Now you have the tools to execute your program and to personalize it to truly change the way you live every day. This is now your way of life. As you enter this way to live, you are now an Efenian.

FIRST WEEK

Even death is not be feared by one who has lived wisely.

—Buddha

1. **Acquire a journal** and write your first thoughts.

Journaling is a trademark of all great leaders and masters.

Action items: Your action plan is to get a journal and start writing your thoughts, ideas, actions, and goals. You will need at least 15 minutes/day for journaling. A good practice is to write in your journal as you get ready to go to sleep (instead of going to sleep with the TV on). Your first writing assignment: You have told that today is your *last day on this earth*, what will your day look like? Write down everything you will do on this day, any regrets, and be as specific as possible in your writing. You are on your way to becoming an Efenian.

2. Evaluate your current fitness level (FQ)

Self-evaluation: Take the FQ (Fitness Quotient) test to evaluate your current state of health and happiness (get a scale of your level) and to find out what areas do you need to start focusing on right away. This test is fairly personal, and no one needs to know your score unless you want them to. Take a picture of your body and record in your journal your current state of health (FQ). Do you have a large percentage of fat, especially around the stomach and buttocks? (Visceral fat). Be as honest as possible with yourself. Write down, also, any current illness, discomfort, and stressors that you are facing at this moment. The more detailed your self-assessment of your current body, the better your plan to change will be. Look at your fat percent, your muscle size and distribution, and your energy level. All the parameters of importance are listed on the FQ test. Go to www.Efenian.com and take the FQ test, record your initial score and make a plan in your journal to start addressing all the factors that you are deficient in. This will be your road map to a new life and to a much better you.

3. Make a list of your current living environment

Action items: Record in your journal your daily eating habits, sleeping habits, any vices (smoking, etc.). To this, you will make a plan to eliminate all the bad habits that are sabotaging your body. Be very specific with the dates and goals (for example, I will stop smoking by Oct 30, 2019). The more specific your goals are, the greater the likelihood of success. Your new diet is a whole food, mostly plant-based diet, and you are getting proper rest, meditation, and exercise. On this list, you will notice things that you are not currently doing, and you will create a plan to start interjecting them into your daily routine. Refer to the Efenian's commitment if you need help in identifying your "bad" habits.

SECOND WEEK

4. Let us start identifying the "stressors" in your life

Action items: In your diary this week, record all the things and or events that make you lose your temper and become stressed. Even if you do not face those events during this week, you can go back to the event where somebody or something made you stressed. Be as specific as possible. Now you can create all tools you need to eliminate all the stress in your life, but we have to start with a detailed list of those items that stress you.

5. Let us continue working with our stressors

This time I want you to focus on physical stressors that are affecting you, and the ones you note in your immediate environment.

Action items: This week you will need to document very specifically all actions to rid of physical stressors identified above. If you have a nagging back pain as one of your physical stressors, then you will need to identify timing and execution of items that will eliminate it (i.e., an exercise routine to make your back stronger for example, etc.).

6. Let us continue working with our stressors, **this time focusing on chemical ones.**

Now focus on any chemical exposure (whether you are eating it, or just by exposing it to the chemical). Chemicals to be on the lookout for would include medicines, processed food, harsh cleaners, and chemical exposure at work and or home.

Action items: List any medication you are currently taking and make a plan to get rid of it. You will need to work with your current doctor and come up with a plan to be rid of any medication. You can eliminate all synthetic medication as the body is self-healing and self-regulating. These will do with medical supervision and with a full understanding of the effect of your medicine and your actions.

7. The last component on your stressor list is **the mental one**

This time you will need to focus on what is making mental stress. Think about the situation in which you feel depressed, hopeless, and gloomy. Record the events that get you there and identify what model or what line of thinking is taking you there. Recall that your reality is what really matters; the rest is just illusion. It is about how you see the world.

Action items: Now that you have a list of mental stressors, let's start identifying action to get rid of each and every one of them. Let's start also listing the positive outlook items that you will be incorporating in your new outlook.

THIRD WEEK

8. We are now entering the zone of **"execution"**

You now must be one hundred percent committed to execution. As an Efenian, you must be a person of action. Now that you are one who does what he says he is going to do, you produce an outcome, you execute.

Action items: Monitor the goals you have set up to this point. Are you executing on those goals or are you coming up with excuses and reasons why you are not doing it? If you selected getting rid of some unnecessary medicines as one of your goals, have you done the steps and actions needed to get it done? Take this time to calibrate all those goals and create a way to very specifically measure each of them. For example, if one of your goals was to improve your physique, write your goal as, I want to reach 12% body fat by Nov. 2022.

9. **The plan** for personal growth

The writing on your journey for this part will entail expanding on our concept in Part One. This time it take a broader perspective with what you have learned so far and redo the exercise where you pretend you only have a few days to live. What will you spend those days doing?

Action items: Write down a list of action items from step #7 and be specific on what you will do to get these completed. By now, the list must include the importance of knowledge and wisdom. And the search for understanding should be one of your top goals. Write down how will you continue to grow intellectually (not just in your field but in all areas of knowledge: math, chemistry, physics, medicine, communication, engineering, etc.).

FOURTH WEEK

10. Create a *nutrition plan*

In this step, you will become a detective and investigate all sources of synthetic chemicals in the food that you are eating. Start by reading every label on the food, the cleaning chemicals you use and that you are exposed to, and any other chemical substance you come into contact with.

Action items: Write down a list of action items on how you will be eliminating exposure to all the substances identified above. Keep specificity in mind and make your timeline to detox realistic and doable.

11. Use *variety* in your nutrition

Consider your current diet. Analyze the nutrient, micronutrient, and phytonutrients, that you are consuming (or not consuming). You should record a typical week of eating and break down all the nutrients that you are consuming. Do not forget to include water as well.

Action items: Write down any deficiencies that you have noticed during your week of study. Research natural products that can provide these nutrients and come up with a plan to incorporate this in your regular diet.

12. Your *fasting plan*

This week, you will start the practice of fasting. You can start slowly by skipping breakfast one day and start journaling how you feel. Be sure to check with your doctors if you have any medical condition. Your goal should be to get to intermittent fasting of a span of sixteen hours without eating. This type of fasting will promote the highest benefits.

Action items: Start your fasting program. Record in your journal the hours you fasted and continue to increase these types of fasts until you can go for sixteen hours without eating (per 24 hrs.). The easiest way to accomplish this is to skip breakfast and stop eating by 8:00 pm. You should eat all your food for the day within an eight-hour period.

13. Let us *start cooking*

Your challenge this week is, if you do not cook, to start cooking. Most people will say they do not have time to cook, but you can prepare a nutritious meal in under an hour. And you can also multitask while cooking and listen to an audiobook, talk to your partner, or any other activity that helps maximize this time.

Action items: Practice cooking. Start with an easy recipe from the internet and start experimenting. Relax and have fun while cooking. Cooking is not about strictly following a recipe. Recipes are suggestions, just like a painting; you can experiment and come up with our own interpretation.

14. Determine your eating nutrient *optimal dosage*

It is now time to continue to analyze your eating habits and to ensure that you are eating a healthy dosage of fats. As many as 30-40% of your daily calories can come from fats as long as these are non-industrial fats.

Action items: Add to your favorite cooking recipe all the fat mentioned above. Make sure that you are eating a handful of mixed, natural made nuts every day. Nuts will not only provide you with healthy fats, but they will improve satiety (which prevents you from reaching for the not so good food, like donuts, or chips).

FIFTH WEEK

15. Formalize *your physical training program*

Your program will have a high aerobic component (like running or playing a sports game) and anaerobic (like weightlifting). These two forms of training will ensure your body looks, feels, and acts to its highest potential.

Action items: Join a gym or any institution that will allow training aerobically and anaerobically. It should be a fun activity to ensure that you will stay with this activity in the long run.

16. *Consolidate your workout* in this section

By now you have been going to your gym and working out on a regular basis. At this time, you need to update your workout schedule and ensure that you are "shocking" the body. The body quickly gets used to a routine. To continue to grow, you must continually update your workout routine. Change it every two to three weeks.

Action items: Update and record your new workout on your journey. Also, you must keep your nutrition up to par to ensure you are progressing towards your goal. You can research different types of workouts on the internet, but ensure you keep varying your workout routine.

SIXTH WEEK

17. Create your own *mind mastery*

Now you have learned about controlling your mind. Think about an instance when you lost control. Analyze those situations and brainstorm ways on how you could have managed the situation better. Consider your daily state of mind: are you positive most of the time? Are you pessimistic? Honestly introspect yourself and write down actions on how to address these items.

Action items: Write down tools to get started mastering your mind. For example, you can use "Breathing techniques" to bring back to control. Brainstorm tools that you can use, and catalog these in your journal.

18. *Live in the present*

Let us ponder your daily affairs. See if you find yourself thinking more about the future, your goals, your new venture, or what you will do when you have enough money to retire. Find out how much time you are spending in the past or the future. If you are spending a large portion of your day on either the past or the future, it is time to gain your life back and start focusing now, the present.

Action items: Write down ideas or triggers that you will use to bring back when you are starting to sail away from the present. It is a matter of relative time spent on the present. It is ok to wonder about the past or imagine your future; the issues become when most of your time is spent in either of these two. More than ninety percent of your time should be spent enjoying the present, living in the present moment, and taking time to smell the roses.

SEVENTH WEEK

19. Making your mental and *social connections*

Do you have a network of support to whom you can go for mental support and sharing? Now, you will look at each one of these networks and identify the members of it. You will need to record each network in your journal and work towards making the bonds between you and your person nodes as strong as possible. To build this bond is a two-way street; it not only benefits you but your partner as well. This relationship should be honest, noble, and sincere. It does not build on parasite relationships where only one is benefiting from the association, but it is built on symbiosis, where both parties benefit.

Action items: Research all your network members and create an action plan to build and strengthen the relationships.

APPENDIX B: FQ—FITNESS QUOTIENT TEST

www.Efenians.com

The FQ index is a guide to measure your overall holistic mental and physical fitness. It focuses on all the parameters needed to obtain a truly happy life. By achieving mental and physical fitness, one is in an optimal state to stay in the happy zone the longest. Happiness is about being in a state of joy, a state of bliss. One moves in and out of this state; hence, the happiest person is the one that stays the longest in this state. In certain parts of the day, one will be happy; then one may get out of this state because of a stressor or any other circumstance. Then one can return to this happy state. Happiness is an aggregate of all these moments. It is not correct to measure happiness by taking a point in time and asking, "Are you happy"? One should take into account a whole lifetime to truly measure happiness. A high FQ person will have the tools needed to stay in the happy zone the longest. Take, for example, a very fit body (athletic body). This person will not suffer from the regular ills that a weak body encounters; hence, his chances of being out of the happy zone due to illness or injury are much less. There is a strong correlation between a high FQ value and being happy; the higher the number, the happier one is

.The detailed criteria are presented on the virtual test at *www.Efenians.com*. One can go to this page and take this test online. The test requires that you complete some physical tests to truly assess the metric. There is some subjectivity on a few metrics but remember: the overall goal of this test is for one to assess one's state of health. This is for your own use and to help you focus on the areas that need the most work, whether these are physical and or mental concerns. The six-pack metric has a much higher weight than any other parameter. The parameter is a key metric to assess overall physical health. If one has a well-defined "six-pack" (abdominal core muscles), it is highly unlikely that this person is not in top physical shape. This metric alone can give an accurate assessment of physical conditioning. The value on the FQ index describes your level of physical and mental fitness.

APPENDIX B

FQ Index Level

Level A - Athlete level (90-100)

A-Level has an athletic physique with a proportional defined muscular structure. A fat percentage of less than 10%. (men), 15% (women). No taking of any medications, drugs, or performance enhancers. Mental toughness and a high level of happiness. They have spent most of their time in a state of flow. The maximum level of holistic health.

Level B: Above Average (80-89)

B-Level has some proportionally defined muscular structure. A fat percentage of less than 15%. (men), (20% women). No taking of any medications. Mentally grounded and relatively high level of happiness

Level C: Average (70-79)

C-Level may show some proportionally defined muscular structure. A fat percentage of less than 20% (men), 25% (women). One may be taking some medications. Emotionally not completely grounded and relatively mid-level of happiness.

Level D: Poor (60-69)

D-Level: Starting to work on body muscular structure. A fat percent higher than 30%. Likely taking medications. Mentally weak and high mood swings. Low level of happiness.

Level F: Need Intervention (0-59)

F-Level has one or more critical areas that need immediate attention.

THE FQ TEST: Calculate your FQ by assigning a point level to each question

HOLISTIC FITNESS CRITERIA (FQ Index Parameters)

1.   Identify your **Stomach Type**: _____

   Pot-Belly: **0-4**   *Average Abs:* **5-9**   *Muscular Abs:* **10-14**   *Athlete (six-pack):* **14-15**

   (Assess your abdominal core muscle strength, flexibility, and definition)

2.   Calculate your **Body Fat %**: _____

   Poor: **0-1**   *Average :* **2-3**   *Ideal:* **4**   *Lean (six-pack):* **5**

   (This metric will also depend on your age and gender)

3.   Identify your **Muscular Composition Type**: _____

   Need Intervention: **0-1**   *Average:* **2**   *Above Average:* **3-4**   *Muscular:* **5**

   (This metric looks at the muscular definition, can one see one's muscular

   definitions?)

4.   Identify your **Flexibility Type**: _____

   Stiff: **0-1**   *Average:* **2**   *Above Average:* **3-4**   *Flexible:* **5**

   (Perform the flexibility tests on the online version of the test to find your

   flexibility level)

5.   Identify your **Strength Type**: _____

    Weak: **0-1**   *Average Strength:* **2-3**   *Strong:* **4-5**

    (Perform the strength tests on the online version of the test to find your strength level)

6.   Identify your **Stamina Type**: _____

    Low Stamina: **0-1**   *Average Stamina:* **2-3**   *Strong stamina:* **4-5**

    (Perform the stamina tests on the online version of the test to find your stamina level)

7.   Rate your **Nutrition Type**: _____

    Poor Nutrition: **0-4**   *Average Nutrition:* **5-7**   *Very Healthy:* **8-10**

    (One will need to evaluate one's current diet and synthetic chemical consumption)

8.   Identify your **Chemical Stressors**: _____

    Toxic: **0-1**   *Mid-Toxic:* **2-3**   *Healthy Exposure:* **4-5**

    (Medications, drugs, etc.) (Some medications) (low toxics chem exposure)

9.   Identify your **Environmental Stressors**: _____

    Toxic: **0-1**   *Mid-Toxic:* **2-3**   *Healthy Exposure:* **4-5**

    (Harsh chemicals, etc.)   (Some heavy cleaners, etc.)   (Low toxics chem exposure)

10.   Identify your **Happiness Level**: _____

    Depress: **0-4**   *Average:* **5-7**   *Happy State:* **8-10**

APPENDIX B

(Levels of gratitude, happiness, laughter, generosity, and social participation)

11.   Identify your **Mental health state**: _____

Negative: **0-1**   *Neutral:* **2-3**   *Positive:* **4-5**

(Levels of positivism, upbeat, and include any mental illness)

12.   Identify your **Relaxation level**: _____

Poor: **0-1**   *Neural:* **2-3**   *Healthy:* **4-5**

(Levels of meditation, relaxation, exercise, overall demeanor)

13.   Identify your **Body Illness Level**: _____

Illness: **0-4**   *Average:* **5-7,**   *Healthy:* **8-10**

(Number of illness, strength of the immune system, and sleeping quality)

14.   Identify your **Pain and Discomfort Levels**: _____

In pain: **0-1**   *Average:* **2-3**   *Healthy:* **4-5**

(Levels of pain, discomforts, lack of sleep, etc.)

15.   Identify your **Body Alignment**: _____

16.   *Misalignment:* **0-1,**   *Average Posture:* **2-3,**   *Correct alignment:* **4-5**

(Levels of pain, discomforts, lack of sleep, etc.)

FQ Score *(Add all points above)*: _____

Add all the points from the above test and compare the score to the above definitions to assess your fitness level. Keep in mind this is a relative measure of fitness and it is meant to help you achieve your goal to be in the best mental and physical condition possible, to live the Efenian's way.

REFERENCES

Author's Note

Neil DeGrasse Tyson, Quote. Twiteer.com, 2013.

Csikszentmihalyi, Mihaly. *Flow: The Psychology of Optimal Experience*. New York: Harper Row, 2009. Print

Prologue

Darwin, Charles: *Origin of Species* (1909).

PART ONE: First Noble Truth

Desmond, Adrian J. (13 September 2002). *"Charles Darwin"*. Encyclopedia Britannica. Retrieved 11 February 2018.

Eldredge N. Darwin's Other Books: *"Red" and "Transmutation" Notebooks, "Sketch," "Essay,"* *and Natural Selection*. PLoS Biol. 2005;3(11): e382. doi:10.1371 / journal.p-bio.0030382.

Glass, Bentley (1959*). Forerunners of Darwin*. Baltimore, MD: Johns Hopkins University Press. p.iv. ISBN 978-0-8018-0222-5.

Chapter 1: Let There be Light

REFERENCES

Bruce Goldstein (2010). Quote: *"The ancient Hindu parable of the six blind men and the elephant...."* Encyclopedia of Perception. SAGE Publications. p. 492. ISBN 978-1-4129-4081-8.

SC.R. Snyder; Carol E. Ford (2013). *Coping with Negative Life Events: Clinical and Social Psychological Perspectives.* Springer Science. p.12. ISBN 978-1-4757-9865-4.

"United States Declaration of Independence," American History, University of Groningen, accessed February 28, 2020, http://www.let.rug.nlusa/documents/1776-1785/the-final-text-of-the-declaration-of-independence july-4-1776.php.

Chapter 2: Home Sapiens

Max D. Cooper and Matthew N. Alder, *The Evolution of Adaptive Immune Systems.* 815-822.

Chapter 3: State of Being

Heather Hasan, *Mendel and the Law of Genetics* (Rosen Publishing, 2004).

R.C. Painter, T.J. Roseboom, and O.P. Bleker (2005*), Prenatal exposure to the Dutch famine and disease in later life: an overview,* Reproductive Toxicology 20 (3), 345-52.

R.L. Jirtle and M.K. Skinner (2007*), Environmental epigenomics and disease susceptibility*, Nature Review Genetics 8, 253-262.

St Clair D., Xu M., Wang P., Yu Y., Fang Y., Zhang F., Zheng X., Gu N., Feng G., Sham P., and He L. *Rates of Adult Schizophrenia Following Prenatal Exposure to the Chinese Famine of 1959-1961.* JAMA 294(5):557-562 (2005).

PART TWO: The second Noble Truth

Storr, Anthony (December 1985). *"Isaac Newton".* British Medical Journal (Clinical Research Edition). 291 (6511): 1779–1784.Doi:10.1136b mj.291.6511.1779. JSTOR 29521701b.

Keynes, Milo (20 September 2008). *"Balancing Newton's Mind: His Singular Behaviour and His Madness of 1692–93".* Notes and Records of the Royal Society of London. 62 (3): 289–300.

Andrew Motte translation of Newton's Principia (1687) Axioms or Laws of Motion.

Chapter 4: As a Matter of Harmony

REFERENCES

"Stress". Merriam-Webster.com. Merriam-Webster, 2019.

Chapter 5: A Pile of Broken Bones

Kondō, Shirō (1985). Primate morphophysiology, locomotor analyses, and human bipedalism. Tokyo: University of Tokyo Press.

Chapter 6:   And Then There Were Pills

Centers for Disease Control and Prevention. Accessed at https://www.cc.gov/chronicdisease/resources/publications /factsheets/diabetes-prediabetes.htm.

Benjamin EJ, Virani SS, Callaway CW, et al. *Heart disease and stroke statistics—2018 update: a report from the American Heart Association.* Circulation. 2018;137:e67–e492.

Centers for Disease Control and Prevention. Accessed at https://gis.cdc.gov/cancer/USCS/DataViz.html.

American Diabetes Association. *Economic Costs of Diabetes in the US in 2017.* Diabetes Care 2018;41(5):917-928. PubMed abstract.

Hurd MD, Martorell P, Delavande A, Mullen KJ, Langa KM. *Monetary costs of dementia in the United States.* N Engl j Med 2013;368(14):1326-34.

Auer, Charles, Frank Kover, James Aidala, Marks Greenwood. *"Toxic Substances: A Half-Century of Progress."* EPA Alumni Association. March 2016.

Trasande, Leonardo (April 19, 2016*). "Updating the Toxic Substances Control Act to Protect Human Health"*. JAMA. 315 (15): 1565–6.
"Toxic Substances Control Act (TSCA)". U. S. Environmental Protection Agency (EPA). Archived from the original on October 16, 2014. Retrieved May 6, 2014.

EarthTalk: Toxic Substances Control Act of 1976? Toilet paper rolls?". Blast magazine.com. January 1, 2011.

"Reducing our exposure to toxic chemicals". Center for Effective Government. Archived from the original on April 29, 2015. Retrieved April 12, 2015.

REFERENCES

David Andrews, Ph.D. Richard Wiles. *Off the Books: Industry's Secret Chemicals,* Environmental Working Group • December 2009.

Hileman, B *"Bisphenol A on Trial."* Chemical & Engineering News Government & Policy, 2007; 85(16). Retrieved April 3, 2009, from http://pubs.acs.org/cen/government/85/8516gov2.html.

Diana Zuckerman, Ph.D., Paul Brown, Brandel France de Bravo, MPH, and Sonia Nagda, MD, MPH, Stephanie Fox-Rawlings, Ph.D., *Are Bisphenol A (BPA) Plastic Products Safe?* National Center for Health Research (2019).

Wikipedia website, https://en.wikipedia.org/wiki/*Glyphosate.*

RED Facts: Glyphosate; EPA-738-F-93-011; US Environmental Protection Agency, Office of Prevention, Pesticides, and Toxic Substances, Office of Pesticide Programs, US Government Printing Office: Washington, DC, 1993.

Crystal Gammon, *Weed-Whacking Herbicide Proves Deadly to Human Cells.* Scientific American Magazine, Environmental Health News, June 23, 2009.

Cressey D (March 25, 2015). *"Widely used herbicide linked to cancer".* Nature. doi:10.1038/nature.2015.17181.

IQVIA Institute Report, *Medicine Use and Spending in the US, A Review of 2018 and Outlook to 2023, May 09, 2019.* www.IQVIAInstitute.org.

Vanessa McMains, Johns Hopkins *study suggests medical errors are third-leading cause of death in US,* HUB, John Hopkins University, 2016.

J Clin Psychiatry. *Prescriptions, Nonmedical Use, and Emergency Department Visits Involving Prescription Stimulants, 2016 Mar; 77*(3): e297–e304., doi: 10.4088/JCP.14m09291.

Merikangas KR, He JP, Burstein M, Swanson SA, Avenevoli S, Cui L, Benjet C, Georgiades K, Swendsen J. Lifetime *prevalence of mental disorders in US adolescents: results from the National Comorbidity Survey Replication--Adolescent Supplement* (NCS-A). J Am Acad Child Adolesc Psychiatry. 2010 Oct;49(10):980-9. PMID: 20855043.

Chapter 7: Mendacious Syndromes

REFERENCES

Ferguson, A. S. "Plato's Simile of Light. (Part II.) The Allegory of the Cave (Continued)". The Classical Quarterly 16, no. 1 (1922): 15–28. JSTOR 63616.

PART THREE: The Third Noble Truth

Rudolph, Susanne Hoeber & Rudolph, Lloyd I. (1983). *Gandhi: The Traditional Roots of Charisma*. University of Chicago Press. ISBN 978-0-226-73136-0.

Sankar Ghose (1991). *Mahatma Gandhi*. Allied Publishers. ISBN 978-81-7023-205-6

Chapter 8: Marathon for Everyone

Cummings, Denis. *"The Myth of Pheidippides and the Marathon."* Finding Dulcinea, 13 Nov.2019 www.findingdulcinea.com /news/sports /2010/April /Myth-of-Pheidippides-and-the-Marathon.html. Accessed 13 Nov. 2019.

Michael Jordan did not make varsity-at first, Newsweek Special Edition 2015.

Eric Zorn, *Without failure, Jordan would be false idol*, Chicago Tribune, 2017.

Mike Reiss, *Bill Belichick not interested in making road struggles a hot topic*, ESPN 2017.

Victoria Hilbert, Monday Motivation: *How Preparation Creates Customer Growth*, Turf Magazine, 2016.

Covey, Stephen R. *The Seven Habits of Highly Effective People*: Restoring the Character Ethic. New York: Simon and Schuster, 1989. Print.

González-Forero, M., Gardner, A. *Inference of ecological and social drivers of human brain-size evolution*. Nature 557, 554–557 (2018).

Chapter 9: A Day on Cloud Nine

Helliwell, J., Layard, R., & Sachs, J. (2018). *World Happiness Report 2018*, New York: Sustainable Development Solutions Network.

Psychology Today, *What is positive psychology?* https://www.psychologytoday.com/us/basics/positive-psychology, 2019.

"Harvard Second Generation Study". Harvard Second Generation Study. Retrieved 26 April 2019.

REFERENCES

Maslow, A.H. "*A theory of human motivation*". Psychological Review. 50 (4): 370–96. (1943).

Deckers, Lambert (2018). *Motivation: Biological, Psychological, and Environmental*. Routledge Press.

Tony Robbins, *Money Master the Game*, Simon and Schuster, Nov 18, 2014.

Lyubomirsky, S. *The how of happiness: a practical guide to getting the life you want.* London: Piatkus, 2013.

Miller, M; Mangano, C; Park, Y; Goel, R; Plotnick, GD; Vogel, RA (2005). "*Impact of cinematic viewing on endothelial function*". Heart. 92 (2): 261–2. doi:10.1136/hrt.2005.061424. PMC 1860773. PMID 16415199.

American Physiological Society. "*Laughter Remains Good Medicine.*" ScienceDaily. ScienceDaily, 17 April 2009.

Wikipedia lead from value (ethics). https://en.wikiversity.org/wiki/Virtues# Moral Virtues_and_Performance_Virtues.
Franklin's 13 Virtues Extract of Franklin's autobiography compiled by Paul Ford.

PART FOUR: The Fourth Noble Truth

"*Hippocrates*". Microsoft Encarta Online Encyclopedia. Microsoft Corporation. 2006. Archived from the original on 2009-10-29.

Garrison, Fielding H. (1966), *History of Medicine*, Philadelphia: W.B. Saunders Company. P94.

Wesley D. Smith. *Hippocrates*. Encyclopedia Britannica. Dec 04, 2019. https://www.britannica.com/biography /Hippocrates.

Chapter 10: A Cocktail of Roses

Attwell L, Kovarovic K, Kendal J., *Fire in the Plio-Pleistocene: the functions of hominin fire use, and the mechanistic, developmental and evolutionary consequences* Anthropol Sci. 2015 Jul 20;93:1-20. doi: 10.4436/JASS.93006. Epub 2015 Mar 19.

Terrence Twomey, *The Cognitive Implications of Controlled Fire Use by Early Humans*. Cambridge Archaeological Journal, 2013.

J. Gowlett, R. Wrangham, *Earliest fire in Africa: Towards the convergence of archaeological evidence and the cooking hypothesis*. Azania Archaeological Research in Africa 48(1):5-30 March 2013.

REFERENCES

DOI: 10.1080/0067270X.2012.756754.

Selby, Anna. (2008). Food through the ages: from stuffed dormice to pineapple hedgehogs. Barnsley, South Yorkshire: Remember When. ISBN 9781781598344. OCLC 853456017.

Sidney Mintz, *Sweetness and Power: The Place of Sugar in Modern History (1985)*.

Katherine Leonard Turner (2014). *How the Other Half Ate: A History of Working-Class Meals at the Turn of the Century*. pp. 56, 142. ISBN 978052027757.

Smith, A.F.; Oliver, G. (2015). *Savoring Gotham: A Food Lover's Companion to New York City*. Oxford University Press, Incorporated. p.24. ISBN 978-0-19-939702-0. Retrieved June 15, 2017.

Gross, Daniel (7 August 1977). *Forbes Greatest Business Stories*. John Wiley & Sons, Inc. pp. 178–192. ISBN 978-0-471-19653-2.

The National Center for Health Statistics. *Health, United States, 2016: with chartbook on long-term trends in health*. https://www.cdc.gov/nchs/data/hus/hus16.pdf#053. Published May 2017. Accessed March 8, 2018.

Murray CJ, Atkinson C, Bhalla K, et al. ; *US Burden of Disease Collaborators. The state of US health, 1990-2010: burden of diseases, injuries, and risk factors*. JAMA. 2013;310:591-608. doi:10.1001/jama.2013.13805.

Song M, Fung TT, Hu FB, et al. *Association of animal and plant protein intake with all-cause and cause-specific mortality*. JAMA Intern Med. 2016;176:1453-1463. doi:10.1001/jamainternmed.2016.4182.

Sánchez-Villegas A, Toledo E, de Irala J, Ruiz-Canela M, Pla-Vidal J, Martínez-González MA. *Fast-food and commercial baked goods consumption and the risk of depression*. Public Health Nutr. 2011;15:424-432. See also, Sommerfield AJ, Deary IJ, Frier BM. *Acute hyperglycemia alters mood state and impairs cognitive performance in people with type 2 diabetes. Diabetes Care*. 2004;27:2335-2340.

Kate Taylor, *These 10 companies control everything you buy*, Business Insider Magazine, Apr 4, 2017.

Bruce Robinson (2011-02-17). *"London: A 'Modern Babylon'"*. bbc.co.uk. Retrieved 2018-04-19.

Rebecca Myers (2013-05-27). *"General History of Women's Suffrage"*. The Independent. Retrieved 2018-04-19.

Robertson, Muriel (1949). *"Marjory Stephenson. 1885–1948"*. Obituary Notices of Fellows of the Royal Society. 6 (18): 562–577. doi:10.1098/rsbm.1949.0013. JSTOR 768940.

Yudkin, John (1944). *"Nutritional Status of Cambridge School-Children"*. British Medical Journal. ii (4362):

REFERENCES

201–214. doi:10.1136/bmj.2.4362.201. PMC 2286012. PMID 20785586.

Yudkin, John (October–November 1946*). "Riboflavin Deficiency in the West African Soldier"*. Journal of Tropical Medicine and Hygiene. 49 (5): 83–87. PMID 20281466.

Yudkin, John (27 July 1957*). "Diet and Coronary Thrombosis"*. The Lancet. 270 (6987): 155–162. doi:10.1016/s0140-6736(57)90614-1. PMID 13450357.

Mandelstam, Joel; J. Yudkin (1952). *"Studies in Biochemical Adaptation. The Effect of Variation in Dietary Protein upon the Hepatic Arginase of the Rat"*. Biochemical Journal. 51 (5): 681–686. doi:10.1042/bj0510681.

Yudkin, John (1964). *"Patterns and Trends in Carbohydrate Consumption and their Relation to Disease"*. Proceedings of the Nutrition Society. 23 (2): 149–162. doi:10.1079/pns19640028.

Sullivan, Patricia (November 24, 2004*). "Ancel Keys, K Ration Creator, Dies"*. The Washington Post. Retrieved 2011-02-05

Ancel Keys (ed*), Seven Countries: A multivariate analysis of death and coronary heart disease, 1980*. Cambridge, Mass.: Harvard University Press. ISBN 0-674-80237-3.

Ian Leslie, *The Sugar Conspiracy*, 2019 Guardian News & Media Limited

Fung, Jason, and Tim Noakes. *The Obesity Code: Unlocking the Secrets of Weight Loss*. Greystone Books, 2016.

Dinu, M; Pagliai, G; Casini, A; Sofi, F (10 May 2017). *"Mediterranean diet and multiple health outcomes: an umbrella review of meta-analyses of observational studies and randomised trials"*. European Journal of Clinical Nutrition. 72 (1): 30–43. doi:10.1038/ejcn.2017.58. PMID 28488692.

Jeanelle Boye; Rui Hai Liu Nutr. *Apple phytochemicals and their health benefits*. Published online 2004 May 12. doi: 10.1186/1475-2891-3-5. PMID: 15140261.

Riccardo Calvani, Anna Picca, Francesco Landi, Maria Rita Lo Monaco, Roberto Bernabei, Emanuele Marzetti. Of Microbes and Minds. *A Narrative Review on the Second Brain Aging*. Frontiers in Medicines, 02 March 2018, https://doi.org/10.3389/fmed.2018.00053.

Chapter 11: Abstemiousness— Life's Gift

Fung, Jason, and Tim Noakes. *The Obesity Code: Unlocking the Secrets of Weight Loss*. Greystone Books, 2016.

REFERENCES

Leonie K Heilbronn, Steven R Smith, Corby K Martin, Stephen D Anton, Eric Ravussin. *Alternate-day fasting in nonobese subjects: effects on body weight, body composition, and energy metabolism* The American Journal of Clinical Nutrition, Volume 81, Issue 1, January 2005, Pages 69–73, https://doi.org/10.1093/ajcn/81.1.69.

Jerry R. Balentine, DO, Melissa Conrad Stöppler, M., *Diabetic Ketoacidosis Causes, Symptoms, Treatment, and Complications.* MediciNet Jan 2020.

Adrienne R.Barnosky, Kristin K.Hoddy, Terry G.Untermana, Krista A.Varady. *Intermittent fasting vs daily calorie restriction for type 2 diabetes prevention: a review of human findings* https://doi.org/10.1016/j.trsl.2014.05.013

Johnstone A., *Fasting for weight loss: an effective strategy or latest dieting trend?* Int J Obes (Lond). 2015 May;39(5):727-33. doi: 10.1038/ijo.2014.214. Epub 2014 Dec 26.

Varady KA, Bhutani S, Church EC, Klempel MC. *Short-term modified alternate-day fasting: a novel dietary strategy for weight loss and cardio protection in obese adults.* Am J Clin Nutr. 2009 Nov;90(5):1138-43. doi: 10.3945/ajcn.2009.28380. Epub 2009 Sep 30

Halagappa VK1, Guo Z, Pearson M, Matsuoka Y, Cutler RG, Laferla FM, Mattson MP. *Intermittent fasting and caloric restriction ameliorate age-related behavioral deficits in the triple-transgenic mouse model of Alzheimer's disease.* Neurobiol Dis. 2007 Apr;26(1):212-20. Epub 2007 Jan 13.

Martin, B., Mattson, M. P., & Maudsley, S. (2006*). Caloric restriction and intermittent fasting: two potential diets for successful brain aging.* Aging research reviews, 5(3), 332–353. doi:10.1016/j.arr.2006.04.002

PART FIVE: The Fifth Noble Truth

Whitehouse, D. (2009). *Renaissance Genius: Galileo Galilei & His Legacy to Modern Science.* Sterling Publishing. ISBN 978-1-4027-6977-1.

O'Connor, J. J., Robertson, E .F. *"Galileo Galilei".* The MacTutor History of Mathematics archive. University of St Andrews, Scotland. Retrieved 24 July 2007

Chapter 12: My New Shiny Exoskeleton

Carrier, D.R.; et al. (Aug–Oct 1984*). "The Energetic Paradox of Human Running and Hominid Evolution".* Current Anthropology. 25 (4): 483–495. doi:10.1086/203165. JSTOR 2742907

REFERENCES

David Sansone. *Ancient Greek civilization*. Wiley-Blackwell, 2003

Harris, H.A. (1964). *Greek Athletes and Athletics*. London: Hutchinson & Co. ISBN 978-0-313-20754-9.

Anderson E, Shivakumar G. *Effects of exercise and physical activity on anxiety*. Front Psychiatry. 2013 Apr 23;4:27. doi: 10.3389/fpsyt.2013.00027. eCollection 2013.

Puetz TW, Flowers SS, O'Connor PJ. *A randomized controlled trial of the effect of aerobic exercise training on feelings of energy and fatigue in sedentary young adults with persistent fatigue*. Psychother Psychosom. 2008;77(3):167-74. doi: 10.1159/000116610. Epub 2008 Feb 14.

Payne C, Wiffen PJ, Martin S. *Interventions for fatigue and weight loss in adults with advanced progressive illness. Cochrane Database* Syst Rev. 2012 Jan 18;1:CD008427. doi: 10.1002/14651858.CD008427.pub2.

Booth, F. W., Roberts, C. K., & Laye, M. J. (2012). *Lack of exercise is a major cause of chronic diseases. Comprehensive* Physiology, 2(2), 1143–1211. doi:10.1002/cphy.c110025

Elizabeth Anderson and Geetha Shivakumar. Effects of Exercise and Physical Activity on Anxiety. JFront Psychiatry. 2013; Published online 2013 Apr 23. Doi: 10.3389/fpsyt.2013.00027 PMCID: PMC3632802

Van Praag, H. *Neurogenesis and exercise: past and future directions*. Neuromolecular medicine (2008)

Müller, S., Preische, O., Sohrabi, H. R., Gräber, S., Jucker, M., Ringman, J. M., & Rossor, M. (2018). *Relationship between physical activity, cognition, and Alzheimer pathology in autosomal dominant Alzheimer's disease. Alzheimer's & Dementia*, 14(11), 1427-1437.

Part Six: The Sixth Noble Truth

Laumakis, Stephen (2008), *An Introduction to Buddhist philosophy*, Cambridge; New York: Cambridge University Press, ISBN 978-0-521-85413-9.

Gombrich, Richard F (1988), *Theravada Buddhism: A Social History from Ancient Benares to Modern Colombo*, Routledge, and Kegan Paul

Narada (1992), *A Manual of Buddhism*, Buddha Educational Foundation, ISBN 978-967-9920-58-1

REFERENCES

"nirvana". Encyclopedia Britannica. Retrieved 22 October 2014.

Chapter 13: Meet Me at The River

Wiley Interdiscip Rev Cogn Sci. 2013 Jan;4(1):33-45. doi: 10.1002/wcs.1206. Epub 2012 Nov 8. Review. PMID: 23529256.

Jon H. Kaas, *The evolution of brains from early mammals to humans First published: 08 November 2012* https://doi.org/10.1002 /wcs.1206.

Benedict Carey (December 6, 2010*). "No Memory, but He Filled In the Blanks"*. New York Times. Retrieved December 5, 2008.

Ibid. Benedict Carey (December 6, 2010*). "No Memory, but He Filled In the Blanks"*. New York Times. Retrieved December 5, 2008.

Freud, Sigmund. *The Standard Edition of the Complete Psychological Works of Sigmund Freud*. Vol. XIX (1999) James Strachey, Gen. Ed. ISBN 0-09-929622-5.

Creswell J.D. (2017). *"Mindfulness Interventions"*. Annual Review of Psychology. 68: 491–516. doi:10.1146/annurev-psych-042716-051139. PMID 27687118.

Bishop, S. R., Lau, M., Shapiro, S. L., Carlson, L., Anderson, N. D., Carmody, J., Devins, G. (2004*). Mindfulness: A proposed operational definition*. Clinical Psychology: Science and Practice, 11, 230–241.

Karen Feldscher, *Study looks at mechanics of optimism in reducing the risk of dying prematurely*, The Harvard Gazette, Dec 7, 2016.

"Meditation". Online Etymology Dictionary, Douglas Harper. 2019. Retrieved 2 February 2019.

Chapter 14: A Kite in The Wind

Jevning; R.K. Wallace; M. Beidebach (1992). *"The physiology of meditation: A review: A wakeful hypometabolic integrated response"*. Neuroscience & Biobehavioral Reviews. 16 (3): 415–24. doi:10.1016/S0149-7634(05)80210-6. PMID 1528528.

Luberto, Christina M.; Shinday, Nina; Song, Rhayun; Philpotts, Lisa L.; Park, Elyse R.; Fricchione, Gregory L.; Yeh, Gloria Y. (2017*). "A Systematic Review and Meta-analysis of the Effects of Meditation on Empathy, Compassion, and Prosocial Behaviors"*. Mindfulness. 9 (3): 708–24. doi:10.1007/s12671-017-

REFERENCES

0841-8. PMC 6081743. PMID 30100929.

Wallace, B. Alan (2006). *The attention revolution: Unlocking the power of the focused mind. Boston: Wisdom.* ISBN 978-0-86171-276-2.c.

Matt J. Rossano (2007). *"Did meditating make us human?".* Cambridge Archaeological Journal. 17 (1): 47–58. Bibcode:2008CArcJ..18.327P.doi:10.1017/S0959774307000054.

Goyal M, Singh S, Sibinga EM, Gould NF, Rowland-Seymour A, Sharma R, Berger Z, Sleicher D, Maron DD, Shihab HM, Ranasinghe PD, Linn S, Saha S, Bass EB, Haythornthwaite JA., *Meditation programs for psychological stress and well-being: a systematic review and meta-analysis.* JAMA Intern Med. 2014 Mar;174(3):357-68. doi: 10.1001/jamainternmed.2013.13018. Review. PMID: 24395196.

Melissa A. Rosenkranza, Richard J.Davidson, Donal G.MacCoon, John F. Sheridand, Ned H. Kalin, Antoine Lutz, A *comparison of mindfulness-based stress reduction and an active control in modulation of neurogenic inflammation, Brain, Behavior, and Immunity.* Volume 27, January 2013, Pages 174-184

Ball MS, Vernon B., *A review on how meditation could be used to comfort the terminally ill.* Palliat Support Care. 2015 Oct;13(5):1469-72. doi: 10.1017/S1478951514001308. Epub 2014 Oct 30.

Gard T., Hölzel BK, Lazar SW, *The potential effects of meditation on age-related cognitive decline: a systematic review, Ann N Y Acad Sci. 2014* Jan;1307:89-103. DOI: 10.1111/nyas.12348.

Sood A., Jones DT. *On mind wandering, attention, brain networks, and meditation.* Explore (NY). 2013 May-Jun;9(3):136-41. doi: 10.1016/j.explore.2013.02.005.

John J., Miller M.D., Ken Fletcher Ph.D., Jon Kabat-Zinn Ph.D. *Three-year follow-up and clinical implications of a mindfulness meditation-based stress reduction intervention in the treatment of anxiety disorders* General Hospital Psychiatry Volume 17, Issue 3, May 1995, Pages 192-200

Carmody, James & Baer, Ruth. (2008*). Relationships between mindfulness practice and levels of mindfulness, medical and psychological symptoms and well-being in a mindfulness-based stress reduction program. Journal of behavioral medicine.* 31. 23-33. 10.1007/s10865-007-9130-7.

Jain FA, Walsh RN, Eisendrath SJ, Christensen S, Rael Cahn B., *Critical analysis of the efficacy of meditation therapies for acute and subacute phase treatment of depressive disorders: a systematic review.* Psychosomatics. 2015 Mar-Apr;56(2):140-52. doi: 10.1016/j.psym.2014.10.007. Epub 2014 Oct 22.

REFERENCES

Institute of Medicine. *Sleep Disorders and Sleep Deprivation: An Unmet Public Health Problem*. Washington, DC: The National Academies Press; 2006.

Martires J, Zeidler M., *The value of mindfulness meditation in the treatment of insomnia.*Curr Opin Pulm Med. 2015 Nov;21(6):547-52. doi:10.1097/MCP.0000000000000207

Galante J, Galante I, Berker MJ, Gallacher J., *Effect of kindness-based meditation on health and well-being: a systematic review and meta-analysis.*, Consult Clin Psychol. 2014 Dec;82(6):1101-14. doi: 10.1037/a0037249. Epub 2014 Jun 30.   Part Seven: The Seventh Noble Truth

Sagan, Carl. *Pale Blue Dot: A Vision of the Human Future in Space*. New York: Random House, 1994.

Sagan, Carl; Head, Tom (2006). *Conversations with Carl Sagan(illustrated ed.)*. Univ. Press of Mississippi. ISBN 978-1-57806-736-7. Also see Poundstone, William (1999). *Carl Sagan: A Life in the Cosmos*. New York: Henry Holt and Company. ISBN 978-0-8050-5766-9. LCCN 99014615. OCLC 40979822.

Davidson, Keay (1999). *Carl Sagan: A Life. New York*: John Wiley & Sons. ISBN 978-0-471-25286-3. LCCN 99036206. OCLC 41580617.

Spangenburg, Ray; Moser, Kit (2004). *Carl Sagan: A Biography*. Westport, CT: Greenwood Publishing Group. ISBN 978-0-313-32265-5. LCCN 2004015176. OCLC 55846272.

Sagan, Carl. *Pale Blue Dot: A Vision of the Human Future in Space*. New York: Random House, 1994.

Chapter 15: A Spider Web

Masi, C.M., Chen, H., Hawkley, L.C., and Cacioppo, J.T. (2011). *A meta-analysis of interventions to reduce loneliness. Personality and Social Psychology Review* 15(3), 219-266.

Kappeler, Peter M.; van Schaik, Carel P. (2002-08-01). *"Evolution of Primate Social Systems"*. *International Journal of Primatology*. 23 (4): 707–740. doi:10.1023/A:1015520830318. ISSN 1573-8604.

Ignoring Genocide (HRW Report - Leave None to Tell the Story: Genocide in Rwanda, March 1999)". www.hrw.org. Retrieved 16 June 2019.

REFERENCES

Ka Hon Chu, Sandra, and Anne-Marie de Brouwer. *"the MEN who KILLED me"*. Herizons 22, no. 4 (Spring 2009): 16. EBSCOhost, MasterFILE Premier p. 16

GLOSSARY

Apoptosis: The death of cells that occurs as a normal and controlled part of an organism's growth or development.

Archaea: Single-celled organisms with structure similar to bacteria. These microorganisms lack cell nuclei and are therefore prokaryotes.

Carcinogen: A cancer-causing or cancer-inciting agent.

Chimeric gene: A gene created by the mixing together of parts from different sources, through the combination of portions of two or more coding sequences.

Chromosome: A threadlike structure of nucleic acids and protein found in the nucleus of most living cells, carrying genetic information in the form of genes.

Cytotoxic: Any agent or process that kills cells.

DNA: Deoxyribonucleic acid is a molecule composed of two chains that coil around each other to form a double helix carrying genetic instructions for the development, functioning, growth, and reproduction of all known organisms and many viruses.

Enzymes: Are both proteins and biological catalysts (biocatalysts). Catalysts accelerate chemical reactions.

Epidemiology: The study and analysis of the distribution (who, when, and where), patterns and determinants of health and disease conditions in defined populations.

Eukaryotes: Organisms whose cells have a nucleus enclosed within membranes, unlike prokaryotes (Bacteria and Archaea), which have no membrane-bound organelles.

Free radicals. An atom, molecule, or ion that has an unpaired valence electron. These unpair electrons make radicals highly chemically reactive. Most organic radicals have short lifetimes.

Gene: A unit of inheritance. It is a sequence of nucleotides in DNA or RNA that encodes the synthesis of a gene product, either RNA or protein.

GLOSSARY

Genetic engineering: Also called genetic modification or genetic manipulation; it is the direct manipulation of an organism's genes using biotechnology.

Genome: The full complement of all genes within the organism.

Incidence: In epidemiology, this is defined as the number of patients who are diagnosed with a disease in a given period of time.

Kinase: An enzyme that catalyzes the transfer of phosphate groups from high-energy, phosphate-donating molecules to specific substrates.

Metastasis: A pathogenic agent's spread from an initial or primary site to a different or secondary site within the host's body.

Mitosis: A part of the cell cycle when replicated chromosomes are separated into two new nuclei. Cell division gives rise to genetically identical cells in which the number of chromosomes is maintained.

Neoplasm, neoplasia: An alternative name for cancer.

Oncogene: A gene that has the potential to cause cancer.

Pathogen: A specific causative agent (such as a bacterium or virus) of disease.

Prevalence: In epidemiology, this is the proportion of a particular population found to be affected by a medical condition (typically a disease or a risk factor such as smoking or seat-belt use).

Prokaryote: A unicellular organism that lacks a membrane-bound nucleus, mitochondria, or any other membrane-bound organelle.

Proteins: Large biomolecules, or macromolecules, consisting of one or more long chains of amino acid residues. Proteins perform a vast array of functions within organisms, including catalyzing metabolic reactions, DNA replication, responding to stimuli, providing structure to cells, and organisms, and transporting molecules from one location to another.

Proto-oncogene: A normal gene that could become an oncogene due to mutations or increased expression.

Retrovirus: A type of RNA virus that inserts a copy of its genome into the DNA of a host cell that it invades, thus changing the genome of that cell.

GLOSSARY

Reverse transcriptase (RT): An enzyme used to generate complementary DNA (cDNA) from an RNA template. Reverse transcriptase is used by retroviruses to replicate their genomes.

Ribonucleic acid (RNA): A polymeric molecule essential in various biological roles in coding, decoding, regulation and expression of genes. RNA and DNA are nucleic acids, and, along with lipids, proteins and carbohydrates, constitute the four major macromolecules essential for all known forms of life.

Stress: In engineering, it is a physical quantity that expresses the internal forces that neighboring particles of a continuous material exert on each other. In psychology, stress is a feeling of strain and pressure.

Strain: In mechanics, strain is a geometrical measure of deformation representing the relative displacement between particles in a material body. In chemistry, a molecule experiences strain when its chemical structure undergoes some stress which raises its internal energy in comparison to a strain-free reference compound.

Virus: A small infectious agent that replicates only inside the living cells of an organism. Viruses can infect all types of life forms, from animals and plants to microorganisms, including bacteria and archaea.

SELECTED BIBLIOGRAPHY

14th Dalai Lama, and Jeffrey Hopkins. *How to Practice: The Way to a Meaningful Life.* London: Rider, 2008. Print.

Anderson E, Shivakumar G., *Effects of exercise and physical activity on anxiety. Front Psychiatry.* 2013.

Anderson, Elizabeth and Geetha Shivakumar. *Effects of Exercise and Physical Activity on Anxiety.* JFront Psychiatry. 2013; Published online 2013 Apr 23.

Andrew, David, and Richard Wiles. *Off the Books: Industry's Secret Chemicals,* Environmental Working Group, December 2009.

Attwell L, Kovarovic K, Kendal J., *Fire in the Plio-Pleistocene: the functions of hominin fire use, and the mechanistic, developmental and evolutionary consequences.* J Anthropol Sci. 2015 Jul 20;93:1-20. doi: 10.4436/JASS.93006. Epub 2015 Mar 19.

Auer, Charles, Frank Kover, James Aidala, Marks Greenwood. *"Toxic Substances: A Half-Century of Progress."* EPA Alumni Association, March 2016.

Balentine, Jerry R. DO, Melissa Conrad Stöppler, M., *Diabetic Ketoacidosis Causes, Symptoms, Treatment, and Complications.* MediciNet, Jan 2020.
Ball MS, Vernon B., *A review on how meditation could be used to comfort the terminally ill.* Palliat Support Care. Epub, 2014.

Bowden, J., & Sinatra, S. *The Great Cholesterol Myth: Why Lowering Your Cholesterol Will not Prevent Heart Disease-and the Statin-Free Plan That Will.* Rockport, MA: Fair Winds Press, 2013.

Buettner, Dan. *The Blue Zones: Lessons for Living Longer From the People Who've Lived the Longest* (First Paperback ed.). National Geographic, 2009.

Calvani, Riccardo, Anna Picca, Francesco Landi, Maria Rita Lo Monaco, Roberto Bernabei, Emanuele Marzetti. Of Microbes and Minds. *A Narrative Review on the Second Brain Aging.* Frontiers in Medicines, 2018.

Campbell, T. Colin., and Howard Jacobson. *Rethinking the Science of Nutrition* BenBella, 2014. Print.

Carey, Benedict (December 6, 2010). *"No Memory, but He Filled In the Blanks".* New York Times, 2008.

Chopra, D. *The ultimate happiness prescription: 7 keys to joy and enlightenment.* London: Rider Books, 2017.

Covey, Stephen R. *The Seven Habits of Highly Effective People: Restoring the Character Ethic.* New York: Simon and Schuster, 1989. Print.

SELECTED BIBLIOGRAPHY

Csikszentmihalyi, *Mihaly. Flow: The Psychology of Optimal Experience.* New York: Harper Row, 2009. Print.

Darwin, Charles: *Origin of Species,* 1909.

Davidson, Keay. *Carl Sagan: A Life.* New York: John Wiley & Sons, 1999.

Deckers, Lambert. *Motivation: Biological, Psychological, and Environmental.* Routledge Press, 2018.

Dietert, Rodney Dietert. *The Human Superorganism: How the Microbiome Is Revolutionizing the Pursuit of a Healthy Life.* New York: Penguin Random House, 2016.

Dinu, M; Pagliai, G; Casini, A; Sofi, F. *"Mediterranean diet and multiple health outcomes: an umbrella review of meta-analyses of observational studies and randomised trials".* European Journal of Clinical Nutrition, 2017.

Feldscher, Karen. *Study looks at mechanics of optimism in reducing the risk of dying prematurely,* The Harvard Gazette, 2016.

Freud, Sigmund. *The Standard Edition of the Complete Psychological Works of Sigmund Freud.* Vol. XIX , 1999.

Fung, Jason, and Tim Noakes. *The Obesity Code: Unlocking the Secrets of Weight Loss.* Greystone Books, 2016.

Gammon, Crystal. *Weed-Whacking Herbicide Proves Deadly to Human Cells.* Scientific American Magazine, Environmental Health News, June 23, 2009.

Ghose, Sankar. *Mahatma Gandhi.* Allied Publishers, 1991.

Glass, Bentley (1959). *Forerunners of Darwin.* Baltimore, MD: Johns Hopkins University Press. 1995.

Gross, Daniel. *Forbes Greatest Business Stories.* John Wiley & Sons, Inc., 1977.

Harris, H.A. *Greek Athletes and Athletics.* London: Hutchinson & Co, 1964.

Hasan, Heather. *Mendel and The Laws Of Genetics.* The Rosen Publishing Group, 2004.

Hurd MD, Martorell P, Delavande A, Mullen KJ, Langa KM. *Monetary costs of dementia in the United States.* N Engl J Med 2013.

Kaas, Jon H. *The evolution of brains from early mammals to humans* First published: 08 November 2012.

Keys, Ancel (ed), *Seven Countries: A multivariate analysis of death and coronary heart disease.* Cambridge, Harvard University Press, 1980.

Kondō, Shirō. *Primate morphophysiology, locomotor analyses, and human bipedalism.* Tokyo: University of Tokyo Press, 1985.

SELECTED BIBLIOGRAPHY

Leslie, Ian, *The Sugar Conspiracy*, 2019 Guardian News & Media Limited.

Lyubomirsky, S. *The how of happiness: a practical guide to getting the life you want*. London: Piatkus, 2013.

Mintz, Sidney, *Sweetness and Power: The Place of Sugar in Modern History*, 1985.

Motte, Andrew. translation of Newton's *Principia* (1687) *Axioms or Laws of Motion*.

Mukherjee, Siddhartha. *The Gene: An Intimate History*, 2019.

Narada, *A Manual of Buddhism*, Buddha Educational Foundation, 1992.

O'Connor, J. J., Robertson, E .F. *"Galileo Galilei"*. *The MacTutor History of Mathematics archive*. University of St Andrews, Scotland. Retrieved 24 July 2007.

Olivelle, Patrick. *Life of the Buddha by Ashva-ghosha* (1st ed.). New York: New York University, 2008.

Polk, Thad A. *The Aging Brain*. Teaching Company, 2010.

Poundstone, William. *Carl Sagan: A Life in the Cosmos*. New York: Henry Holt and Company, 1999.

Rankin, Lissa. *Mind over medicine. Scientific proof that you can heal yourself*. London: Hay House, 2013. Print.

Robbins, Tony, *Mastering the game*, Simon and Schuster, Nov 18, 2014.

Robbins, Tony. *Unshakeable: Your Financial Freedom Playbook*. Simon & Schuster, 2018. Print.

Rudolph, Susanne Hoeber & Rudolph, Lloyd I. *Gandhi: The Traditional Roots of Charisma*. University of Chicago Press, 1983.

Sagan, Carl. *Pale Blue Dot: A Vision of the Human Future in Space*. New York: Random House, 1994.

Sagan, Carl; Head, Tom. *Conversations with Carl Sagan illustrated ed.)*. Univ. Press of Mississippi, 2006.

Sansone, David Sansone. *Ancient Greek civilization*. Wiley-Blackwell, 2003.

Selby, Anna. *Food through the ages: from stuffed dormice to pineapple hedgehogs*. Barnsley, South Yorkshire: Remember When, 2008.

Smith, A.F.; Oliver, G. (2015). *Savoring Gotham: A Food Lover's Companion to New York City*. Oxford University Press, 2017.

Snyder, SC.R.; Carol E. Ford. *Coping with Negative Life Events: Clinical and Social Psychological Perspectives*. Springer Science, 2013.

SELECTED BIBLIOGRAPHY

Spangenburg, Ray; Moser, Kit (2004). *Carl Sagan: A Biography*. Westport, CT: Greenwood Publishing Group, 2004.

Turner, Katherine Leonard (2014). *How the Other Half Ate: A History of Working-Class Meals at the Turn of the Century*, 2014.

Van Praag, H. *Neurogenesis and exercise: past and future directions*. Neuromolecular medicine, 2008.

Wallace, B. Alan. *The attention revolution: Unlocking the power of the focused mind*. Boston: Wisdom, 2006.

Whitehouse, D. (2009). *Renaissance Genius: Galileo Galilei & His Legacy to Modern Science*. Sterling Publishing.